Manual of Primary Care Dermatology

D. Kishore Yellumahanthi

Manual of Primary Care Dermatology

Springer

D. Kishore Yellumahanthi
Physician
Huntsville Hospital
Huntsville, Alabama, USA

Clinical Associate Professor
Department of Family Medicine
University of Alabama at Birmingham
Huntsville Regional Medical Campus
Huntsville, Alabama, USA

Adjunct Assistant Professor
of Dermatology
Department of Dermatology
Vanderbilt University School of Medicine
Nashville, Tennessee, USA

Adjunct Faculty
Department of Family Medicine
University of South Alabama
Mobile, Alabama, USA

ISBN 978-3-031-68405-0 ISBN 978-3-031-68406-7 (eBook)
https://doi.org/10.1007/978-3-031-68406-7

This Springer imprint is published by the registered company Springer Nature Switzerland AG
The registered company address is: Gewerbestrasse 11, 6330 Cham, Switzerland

Preface

This book comprises mainly common dermatological cases that can be managed in primary care. In order to tailor the book specifically to the needs of the practicing primary care provider, only clinically relevant aspects of the diseases are discussed in the book. The objective of the book is to aid primary care providers in making sure the diagnosis of the common dermatological conditions seen and that can be managed in primary care are not missed.

The differential diagnosis is mainly discussed based on the body part that is affected with skin ailment. This type of compilation makes it easy for readers in aiding in knowing the diagnosis of their patient's skin condition as what all they need to do is just to refer to that part of the book that discusses the relevant part of the body, for instance, scalp, face or upper extremity.

I hope the book meets its objective and you will enjoy reading this book.

D. Kishore Yellumahanthi, MD, MPH
Physician, Huntsville Hospital
Huntsville, Alabama, USA

Clinical Associate Professor
Department of Family Medicine
University of Alabama at Birmingham
Huntsville Regional Medical Campus
Huntsville, Alabama, USA

Adjunct Assistant Professor of Dermatology
Department of Dermatology
Vanderbilt University School of Medicine
Nashville, Tennessee, USA

Adjunct Faculty
Department of Family Medicine
University of South Alabama
Mobile, Alabama, USA

Acknowledgements

First and foremost, I thank all my patients who had given me their consent to be photographed and to be a part of this book. If not for them, this book would have been incomplete.

My sincere thanks to my colleagues and staff at Family Medicine of Huntsville and at Huntsville Hospital Physician Care, Airport Road, Huntsville, Alabama, USA, for their continued cooperation.

My sincere appreciation to Mr. Grant Weston and other Springer Nature's team for making sure 'my idea' is transformed into print and electronic media and reached the intended readers globally.

Last but not least, I am thankful to my wife, Lata and my children Shushruth and Prithvi for their support during this time to make sure I have time to produce this book.

Contents

About the Author

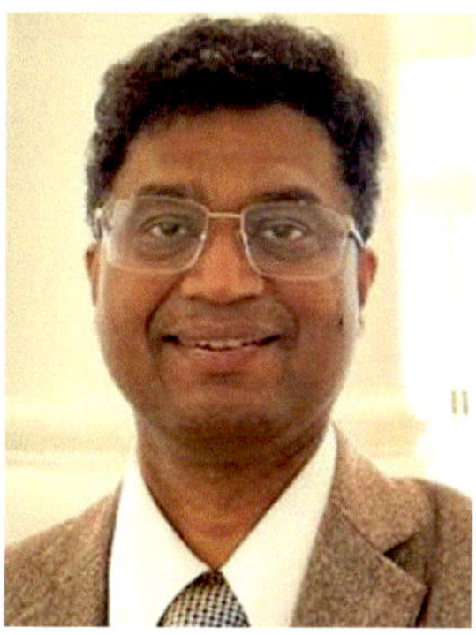

Dr. D. Kishore Yellumahanthi, MD, MPH, FAAFP Currently works as Physician for Huntsville Hospital in Huntsville, Alabama. He practices primary care with a strong affinity for dermatological diseases.

He is a Clinical Associate Professor at the Department of Family Medicine, University of Alabama at Birmingham (UAB), Huntsville Regional Medical Campus, Alabama and Adjunct Assistant Professor of Dermatology at Vanderbilt University of School of Medicine, Nashville, Tennessee. He also serves as Adjunct Faculty in the Department of Family Medicine at University of South Alabama, Mobile, Alabama.

Dr. Yellumahanthi's educational background is unique in that he has expertise and formal training in both Dermatology and Family Medicine. He has completed Residency in Family Medicine at the University of Alabama, Tuscaloosa, Alabama. Prior to that, he had also completed postgraduate training in MD Dermatology (Equivalent to Residency in Dermatology) in India and worked as Consultant Dermatologist for few years.

Dr. Yellumahanthi has published in reputed journals and presented his scientific work at several national and international conferences including American Academy of Dermatology (AAD) Annual Meetings. His research work has won several accolades including the *'Best Scientific Paper'* (Southern Surgical Association Annual Meeting, Palm Beach, Florida), and *'Outstanding Research Award'* (Residency, University of Alabama, Tuscaloosa, Alabama).

Dr. Yellumahanthi enjoys sharing his knowledge and expertise with primary care providers, trainees and the community through guest lectures.

He was invited as guest speaker at various levels including the American Academy of Family Physicians (AAFP) Scientific Assembly.

Dr. Yellumahanthi is a distinguished Fellow of *American Academy of Family Physicians* and *American Contact Dermatitis Society. He is a member of International Dermoscopy Society and National Psoriasis Foundtion.*

Chapter 1
Morphology of Skin Lesions

Abstract In order to be able to diagnose dermatological diseases, knowing the descriptive terminology is useful. Also, being able to precisely describe skin lesions helps in communication among healthcare providers. Included in this chapter are description of the morphology of the skin lesions that are commonly encountered.

Keywords Macule · Patch · Atrophy · Purpura · Excoriation · Erosion · Crust · Lichenification · Plaque · Blister · Vesicle · Bulla · Papule

Macule: A circumscribed discoloration of the skin of size less than 1 cm that is even with the surface level of the surrounding skin (Fig. 1.1).

Patch: A circumscribed discoloration of the skin of size equal to or greater than 1 cm that is even with the surface level of the surrounding skin (Fig. 1.2).

Papule: A circumscribed elevated solid skin lesion that is less than 1.0 cm in size (Fig. 1.3).

Plaque: A plaque is usually formed by coalescence of papules. It is a raised solid plateau like skin lesion, that has a diameter of 1 cm or more (Fig. 1.4).

Vesicles and Bullae: Vesicle is a visible fluid filled skin lesion that is less than 1 cm in diameter (Fig. 1.5). Bullae are similar to vesicles except that size is greater than or equal to 1 cm.

See tense bulla in Fig. 1.6 and flaccid bulla in Fig. 1.7.

Pustule: A pustule is a circumscribed raised skin lesion containing visible pus (Fig. 1.8).

Nodule: A solid or cystic mass in the skin which can either be palpated or found as an elevation during inspection of the skin. It is more than 1 cm in diameter (Fig. 1.9).

Ulcer of the skin: A loss of epidermis and at least a part of the underlying dermis (Fig. 1.10).

D. K. Yellumahanthi, *Manual of Primary Care Dermatology*,
https://doi.org/10.1007/978-3-031-68406-7_1

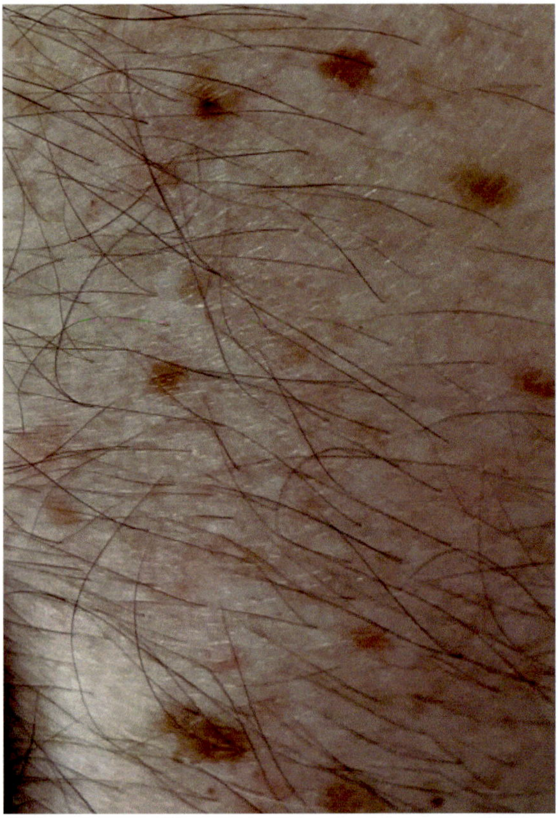

Fig. 1.1 Multiple macules

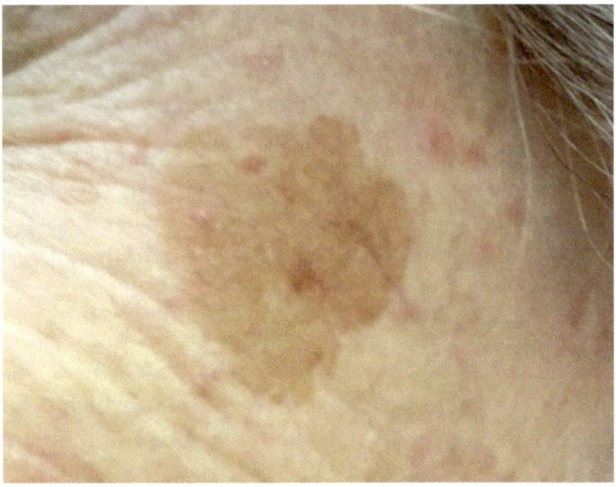

Fig. 1.2 Patch

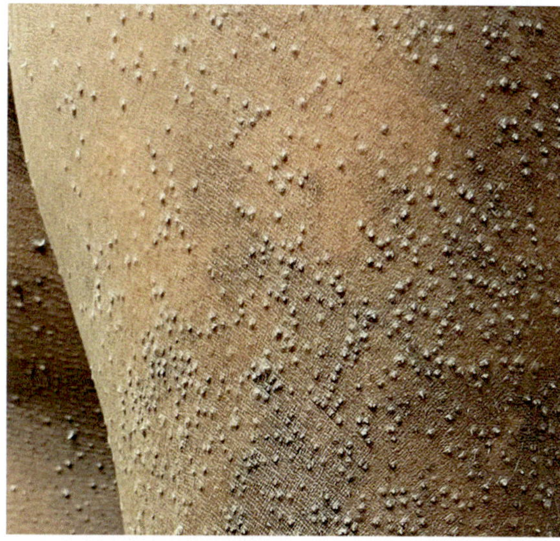

Fig. 1.3 Multiple papules

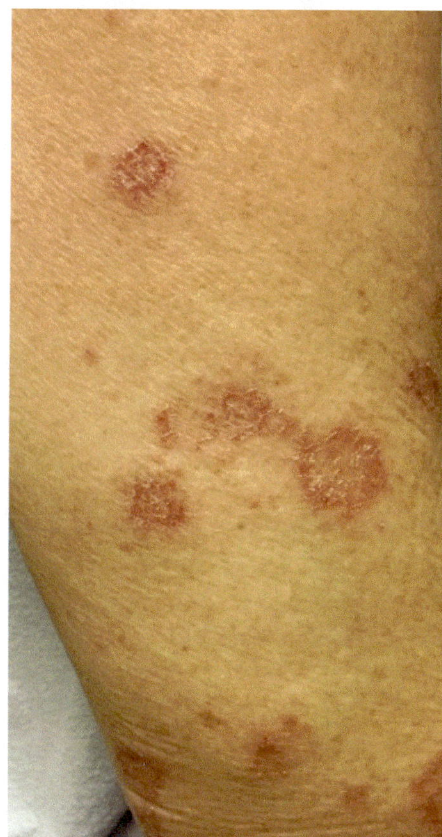

Fig. 1.4 Plaques

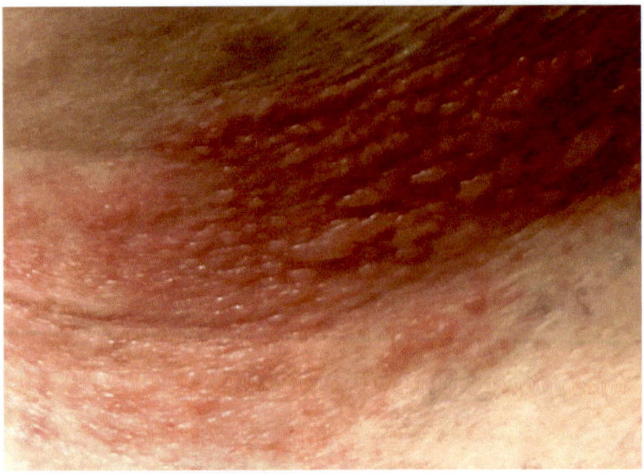

Fig. 1.5 Vesicles

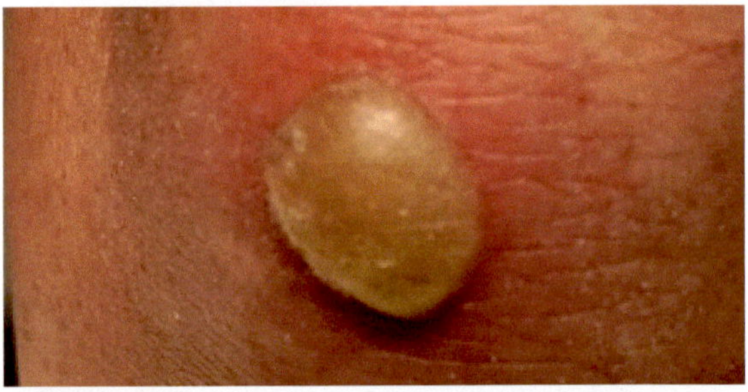

Fig. 1.6 Tense bulla

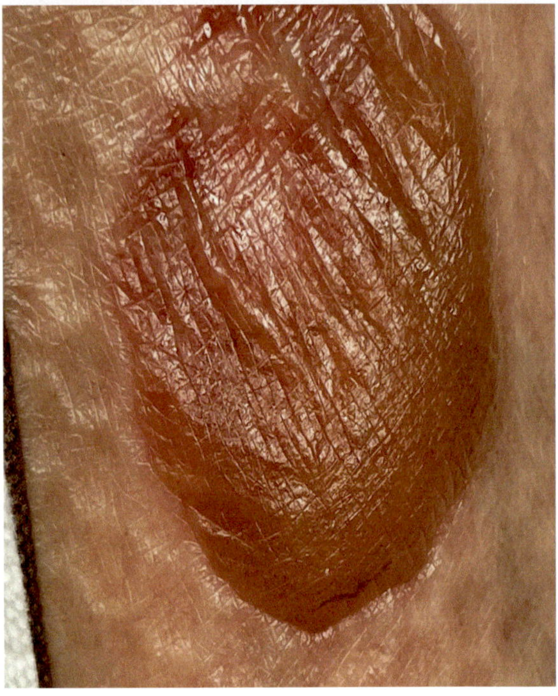

Fig. 1.7 Flaccid bulla

Fig. 1.8 Pustules

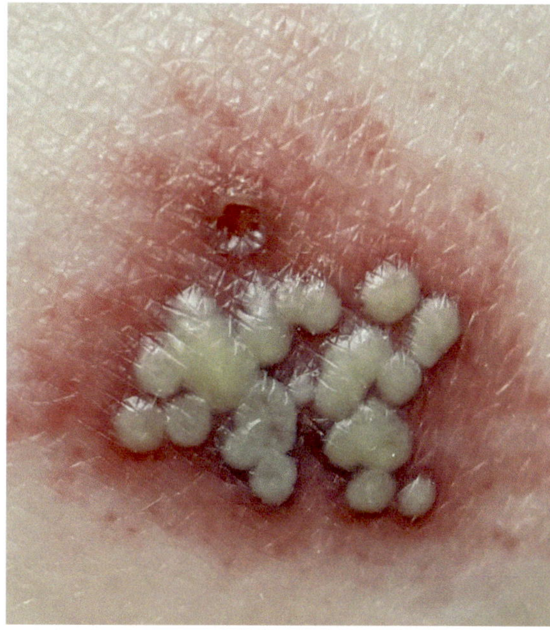

Fig. 1.9 Nodule

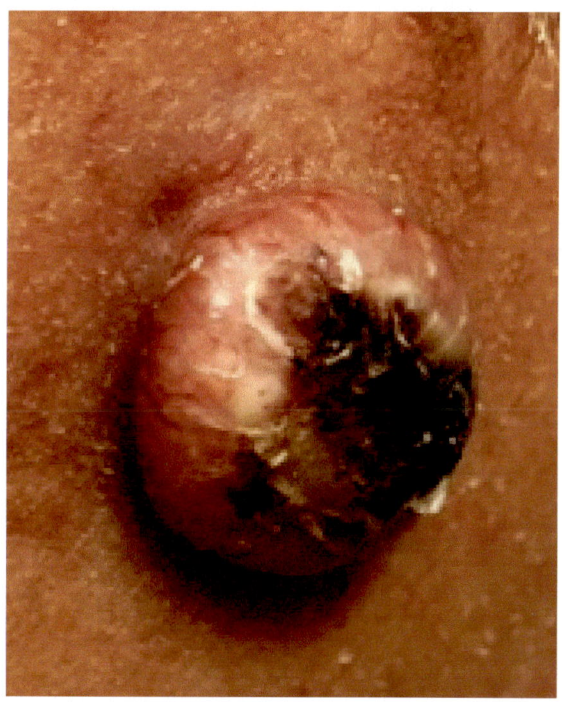

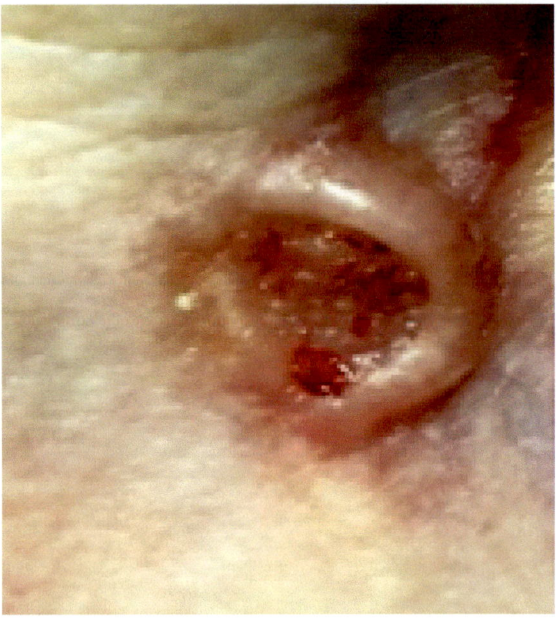

Fig. 1.10 Ulcer

Wheal: A wheal is an edematous, well-defined papule or plaque seen in urticaria that usually lasts less than 24 hours. It is also called hive (Fig. 1.11).

Petechiae: Petechiae are non-blanchable spots on skin or mucosa that measure less than 2 mm in size (Fig. 1.12).

Purpura: A purpura is a non-blanchable spot on skin or mucosa that measure 2 mm or greater in size (Fig. 1.13).

Scale: A scale is a flat plate or flake of stratum corneum (Fig. 1.14).

Excoriations: Excoriation is a loss of skin usually in a linear fashion occurring commonly as a result of scratching (Fig. 1.15).

The presence of excoriations suggests that the skin condition that patient has is probably very itchy.

Erosion and Crust: Erosion: Loss of only epidermis without an associated loss of underlying dermis (Fig. 1.16).

Crust: It is dried fluid such as blood, serum or pus or a combination on the skin's surface (Fig. 1.17).

Lichenification: Lichenification is featured by thickening and accentuation of the skin creases. It is usually a result of repeated scratching or rubbing of the skin (Fig. 1.18).

Atrophy: Atrophy of the epidermis appears as 'cigarette-paper' like wrinkling. Atrophy of the dermis causes a depression in the lesion (Fig. 1.19).

Fissure: A fissure is formed due to dryness or excessive tension of the underlying tissue. It manifests as loss of continuity of the skin or mucosa in a linear fashion (Fig. 1.20).

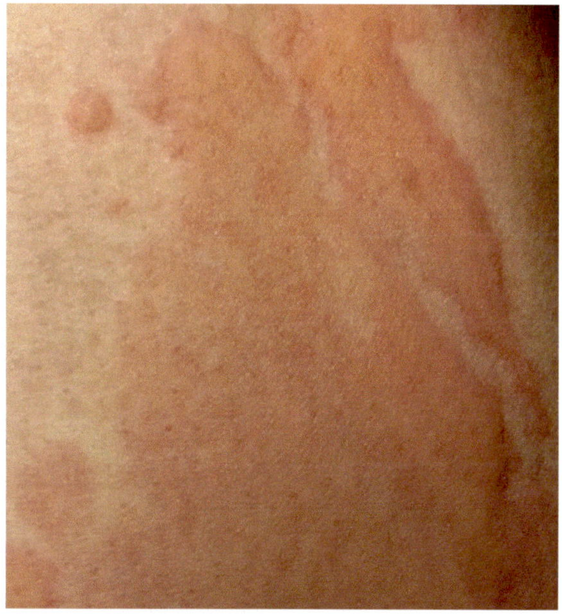

Fig. 1.11 Wheal

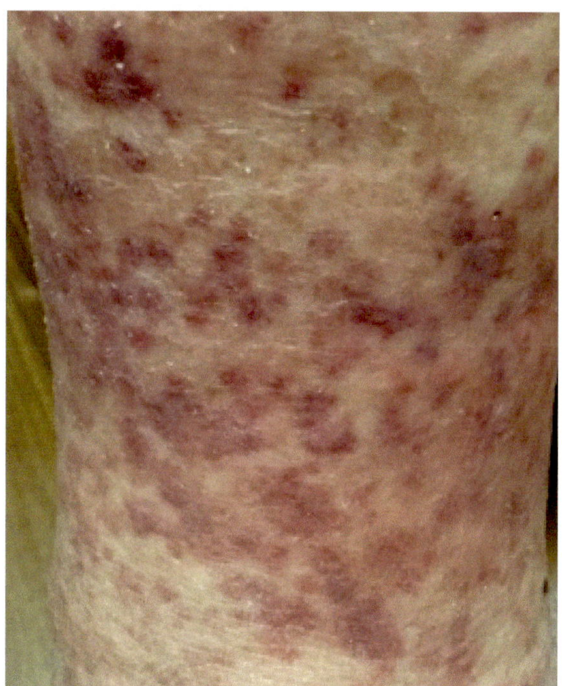

Fig. 1.12 Petechi

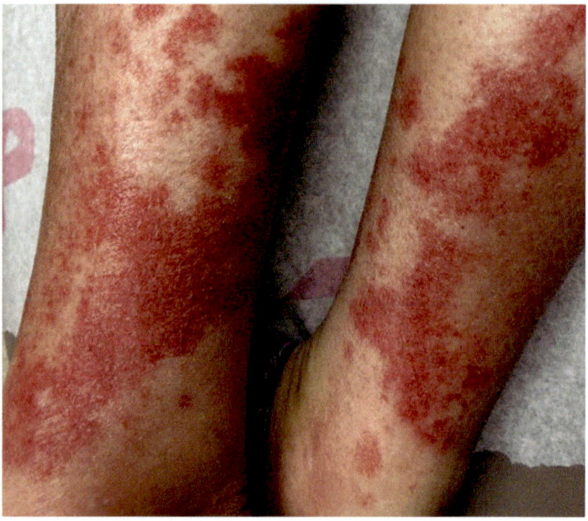

Fig. 1.13 Purpura

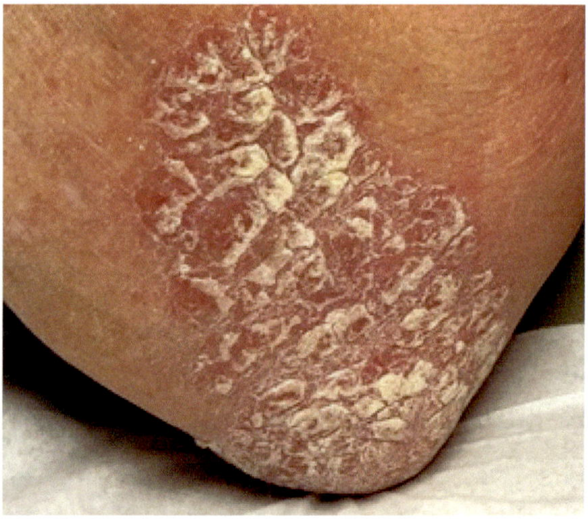

Fig. 1.14 Plaque of psoriasis adherent with scales

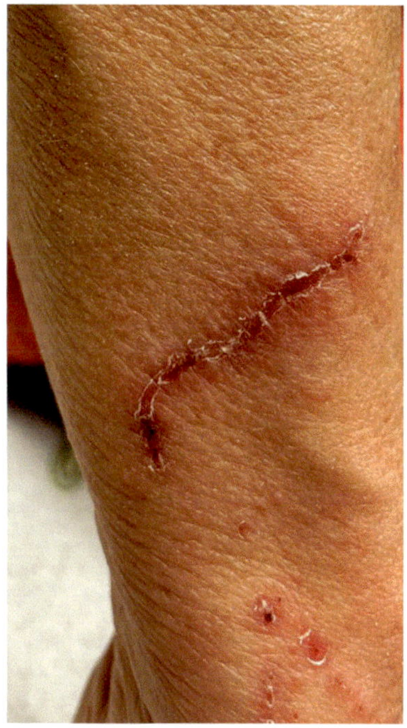

Fig. 1.15 Excoriation. See the linear lesion

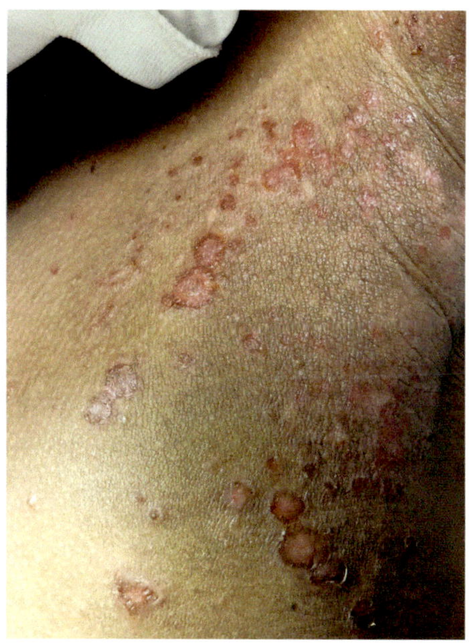

Fig. 1.16 Multiple erosions

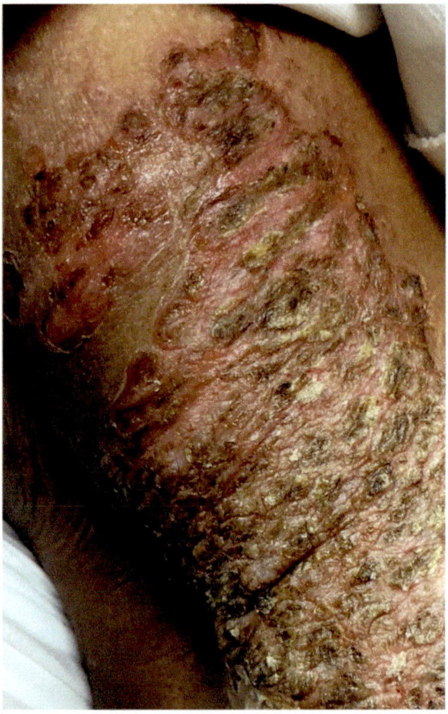

Fig. 1.17 Several crusts

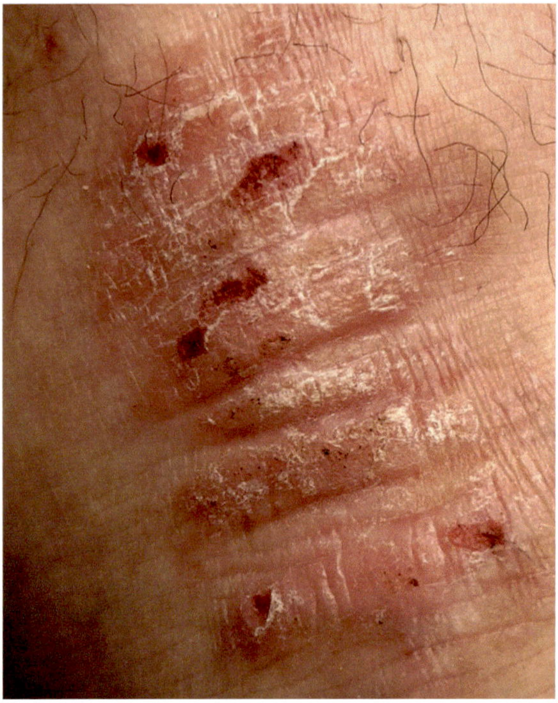

Fig. 1.18 Lichenified plaque

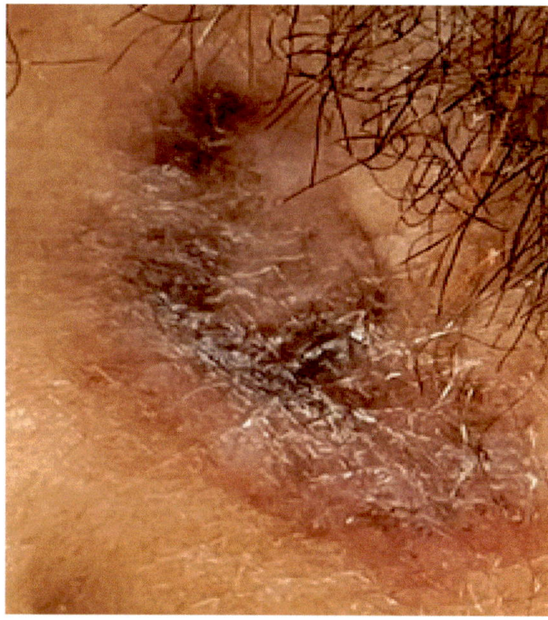

Fig. 1.19 Dermal atrophy

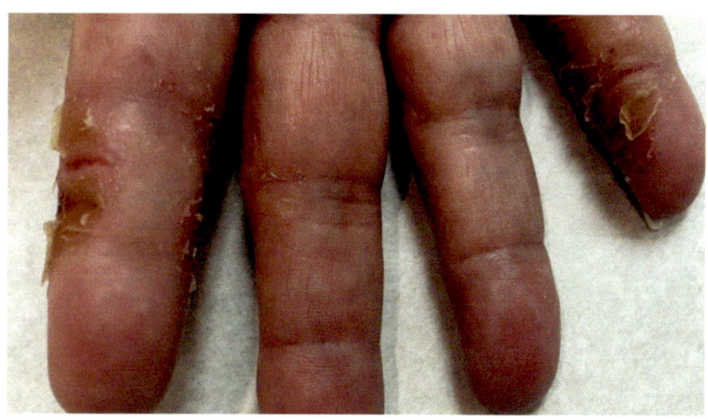

Fig. 1.20 Fissure seen on the middle third of index finger

Bibliography

Amerson EH, Burgin S, Shinkai K. Fundamentals of clinical dermatology: morphology and special clinical considerations. In: Kang S, Amagai M, Bruckner AL, Enk AH, Margolis DJ, McMichael AJ, Orringer JS, editors. Fitzpatrick's Dermatology, 9e. McGraw-Hill Education; 2019.

McGrath A, Barrett MJ. Petechiae [Internet]. PubMed. Treasure Island (FL): StatPearls Publishing; 2020. Available from https://www.ncbi.nlm.nih.gov/books/NBK482331/.

Wheal [Internet]. www.dermweb.com. Available from http://www.dermweb.com/morphology/wheal1.htm.

Chapter 2
Topical Corticosteroids

Abstract Topical steroids are very commonly used by the dermatologists and other providers who manage skin diseases. Unfortunately, not much training is given to the primary care trainees during their respective curriculum about its usage. As a result, most primary care providers are hesitant to use them. Topical steroids need to be used with caution and prudence. If inappropriately a high potent one is used, it can cause unnecessary side effects of topical steroids such as atrophy, telengectasia, hypopigmentation, hypertrichosis. On the other hand, using a topical steroid that is therapeutically subpotent is not going to be helpful to the patient. This chapter provides some practical tips regarding their usage.

Keywords Topical steroids · Potency of steroids · Side effects of steroids · Super potent or ultra potent steroid · High potent steroid · Moderate potent steroid

2.1 Topical Corticosteroids

Topical steroids are an integral part of a dermatologist's therapeutic armamentarium. The topical steroids used in dermatology can be broadly divided on the basis of their potency into super- or ultrapotent, high potent, mid-potent and low potent (Table 2.1).

2.1.1 The Common Factors That Determine the Usage of Appropriate Topical Steroid

– The age of the patient, for instance, in the infants it is prudent to use only lower to mid-potent topical steroids. So, also in the very elderly as their skin is fragile.

– Body site: For instance, on the face, low potent topical steroids are usually recommended.

D. K. Yellumahanthi, *Manual of Primary Care Dermatology*,
https://doi.org/10.1007/978-3-031-68406-7_2

Table 2.1 Potency ranking of selected topical corticosteroid preparations (Topical Steroid Potency Chart)

Super (ultra) potent
Clobetasol propionate 0.05% ointment
Augmented betamethasone dipropionate 0.05% ointment
Halobetasol propionate 0.05%
Fluocinonide 0.1% cream
High potent
Betamethasone dipropionate 0.05% ointment
Desoximetasone 0.25% ointment
Fluocinonide 0.05% ointment
Triamcinolone acetonide 0.5% ointment
Moderate potent
Hydrocortisone valerate 0.2% ointment
Hydrocortisone butyrate 0.1% ointment
Desoximetasone 0.05% cream
Betamethasone valerate 0.1% cream
Triamcinolone acetonide 0.1% ointment
Fluocinolone acetonide
Low potent
Desonide 0.05% cream
Hydrocortisone 2.5% cream

– The thickness of the skin lesion: The thicker the lesion, usually the potent the topical steroid needed.

– The type of skin disease for which it is being used. For instance, psoriasis usually requires superpotent topical steroid.

For a non-dermatologist, given that there are so many topical steroids of various potency, often it becomes challenging to choose the appropriate one. The following practical tips are provided to address that challenge:

– Familiarize oneself with one topical steroid in each of the potency group. For instance, among superpotent, Clobetasol propionate 0.05% ointment, among the high potent, betamethasone dipropionate 0.05% ointment, among mid-potent hydrocortisone valerate 0.2% ointment and desonide 0.05% cream if you want to use anything of lower potency than hydrocortisone valerate 0.2% ointment.

– When to use super potent topical steroids?
  Given that superpotent topical steroids are the most potent steroids and have potential for causing sometimes irreversible side effects, care should be exercised in prescribing them. To avoid injudicious use of these steroids, it may be best to keep in mind a few selective scenarios when one wants to use them. A couple of common scenarios to remember are below.

  1. Any lesions on palms and soles
  2. Psoriasis anywhere on the body except face.
     (Although one can use superpotent steroids for multiple other scenarios, for simplicity, only two common indications are mentioned here)

- For any lesions on the face, use low potent steroids such as desonide 0.05% cream

- In infants, try to minimize usage to desonide 0.05% cream regardless of the body site or high.

- Elderly patients usually have thin skin, which allows for increased penetration of topical glucocorticoids. Similar precautions used in the treatment of infants, should be exercised while treating elderly patients.

2.1.2 *Ointments, Creams and Lotions*

- Is the efficacy of ointment of a drug is same as its cream form?
  In general, ointments tend to stick to the body better than creams. As a result, the ointment form of the same medication tends to be more effective than its cream form (Butala and Paller 2022).

- Creams are less sticky and therefore tend to be more acceptable from cosmetic point of view. They are preferred for moist lesions and also in intertriginous areas (Hengge et al. 2006).

- Lotions are most appropriate in hairy areas.

- Suspensions and foams also work in hairy areas.

2.1.3 *Adverse Effects of Topical Steroids*

- These include but not limited to atrophy (both dermal and epidermal), telengectasia, hypopigmentation, hyperpigmentation, striae, purpura and hypertrichosis (Hengge et al. 2006).

- Contact dermatitis to topical steroids can also occur (Bircher et al. 1995; Lutz and El-Azhary 1997).

- Atrophy is the most common adverse effect of topical corticosteroid therapy (Ponec et al. 1979).

- While atrophy of the epidermis appears as "cigarette-paper" like wrinkling, atrophy of the dermis manifests as a depression in the lesion.

– Although topical glucocorticosteroids can also cause systemic side effects, they are less common than local side effects (Robertson and Maibach 1982; Lagos 1998).

– Ocular hypertension, cataract, glaucoma, perioral dermatitis and steroid induced acne and rosacea are some of the examples of non-local adverse effects of topical steroids. Hypothalamic–pituitary–adrenal (HPA) axis suppression can also occur when wide areas are involved in applying (Zhao et al. 2023).

Bibliography

Bircher AJ, Thürlimann W, Hunziker T, Pasche-Koo F, Hunziker N, Perrenoud D, et al. Contact hypersensitivity to corticosteroids in routine patch test patients. Dermatology. 1995;191(2):109–14.

Butala S, Paller AS. Optimizing topical management of atopic dermatitis. Ann Allergy Asthma Immunol. 2022;128(5):488–504.

Hengge UR, Ruzicka T, Schwartz RA, Cork MJ. Adverse effects of topical glucocorticosteroids. J Am Acad Dermatol. 2006;54(1):1–15.

Lagos M. Frequency of application of topical corticosteroids: an overview. Br J Dermatol. 1998;139(5):763–6.

Lutz ME, El-Azhary RA. Allergic contact dermatitis due to topical application of corticosteroids: review and clinical implications. Mayo Clin Proc. 1997;72(12):1141–4.

Ponec M, Kempenaar JA, Der V, Bachra BN. Effects of glucocorticosteroids on cultured human skin fibroblasts-IV. Biochem Pharmacol. 1979;28(18):2777–83.

Robertson DB, Maibach HI. Topical corticosteroids. Int J Dermatol. 1982;21(2):59–67. Available from https://pubmed.ncbi.nlm.nih.gov/6461612/.

Topical Steroid Potency Chart [Internet]. www.psoriasis.org. Available from https://www.psoriasis.org/potency-chart/.

Zhao S, Hwang A, Miller C, Lio P. Safety of topical medications in the management of paediatric atopic dermatitis: an updated systematic review. BJCP Br J Clin Pharmacol/br J Clin Pharmacol. 2023;89(7):2039–65.

Chapter 3
Papulosquamous Disorders (Skin Disorders with Scales)

Abstract This chapter provides an overview of the common papulosquamous disorders such as psoriasis, lichen planus and pityriasis rosea. It also includes other conditions such as cutaneous lupus that can present with scaly lesions and can come in the differential diagnosis of paplosquamous disorders. The chapter discusses mainly from their clinical perspective. It provides details about the clinical presentation of these conditions and ways to diagnose them; when feasible it provides clinical information regarding how to diagnose them clinically. It also discusses their treatment options and where appropriate the circumstances as to when the patients need to be referred to the dermatologist.

Keywords Psoriasis · Lichen planus · Pityriasis rosea · Cutaneous lupus erythematosus · Discoid lupus erythematosus · Subacute lupus erythematosus

The following is not the comprehensive list of all those dermatological conditions that manifest with scales or papulosquamous lesions. However, the following conditions that are listed below needs to be ruled out as these conditions, if are diagnosed, can be managed in primary care. Please note that any of these conditions, based on the extent of involvement and severity, might have to be referred to a dermatologist, at any point.

– Psoriasis

– Lichen Planus

– Pityriasis Rosea

– Seborrheic Dermatitis

– Subacute Cutaneous Lupus Erythematosus

D. K. Yellumahanthi, *Manual of Primary Care Dermatology*,
https://doi.org/10.1007/978-3-031-68406-7_3

- Please note infections, tinea corporis & pityriasis versicolor also have some scaling and at times can mimic papulosquamous disorders.

3.1 Psoriasis

- Psoriasis is a chronic, common, papulosquamous skin disorder. The exact etiology is unknown. Several factors such as genetic susceptibility, stress, obesity, smoking, alcohol consumption and streptococcal infection have been discussed in its etiology and Interleukin (IL)-17 and IL-23 are incriminated as key drivers in its pathogenesis (Griffiths et al. 2021).

- Psoriasis can manifest as different morphological forms. Chronic plaque form (Psoriasis vulgaris) and Guttate Psoriasis are the common ones seen in Primary care.

- Based on the site of involvement, the variants of psoriasis include flexural or inverse psoriasis, sebopsoriasis, palmoplantar psoriasis and nail psoriasis (Griffiths et al. 2021).

3.1.1 Psoriasis Vulgaris

Psoriasis vulgaris is the most common type of Psoriasis.

- Onset is usually insidious

- Itching none or minimal

- Upon cutaneous examination, well demarcated, erythematous plaques covered with thick, silvery scales are noticed. Size of the lesions can vary from pinpoint papules to large plaques (Fig. 3.1).

- Often when a psoriatic scale is being removed, it causes damage to the underlying dilated capillaries and causes bleeding—Auspitz sign.

- The lesions are usually distributed symmetrically and involve predominantly the extensor aspects of the body such as back of elbows, extensors of forearms, front of the knees and back of the trunk.

- Scalp may be involved.

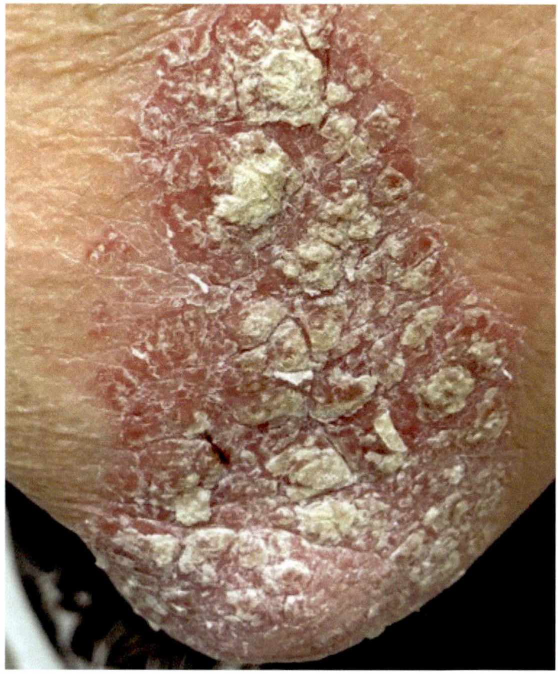

Fig. 3.1 Psoriatic vulgaris

- No mucosal lesions are noted.
- Nail changes can be found in up to 40% of patients (Gudjonsson et al. 2006).

  They include pitting, onycholysis (separation of the nail plate from the nail bed), oil spots (Orange–yellow discoloration of the nail bed), dystrophy and subungual hyperkeratosis.
- Among these, oil spotting is considered to be more specific for psoriasis (Gudjonsson and Elder 2019).
- The involvement of nails, particularly onycholysis, doubles the risk of psoriatic arthritis (Wilson et al. 2009).
- Psoriatic arthritis occurs in about 40% of patients (Gudjonsson and Elder 2019).
- **Diagnosis**: Psoriasis can be usually diagnosed based on clinical features and its typical distribution. Biopsy is indicated to establish the diagnosis, when clinical history and examination is not diagnostic.

Management

- Patients need to be counseled on the chronic nature of the condition and that it can be associated with remissions and exacerbations.

- Topical and systemic therapies are available.

- Topical therapy: Topical super potent corticosteroids such as clobetasol propionate 0.05% ointment are the first line of agents. Topical calcipotriene (vitamin D3 analogue), tazarotene, salicyclic acid, coal tar and emolients are also beneficial. Roflumilast 0.3% cream is a phosphodiesterase 4 inhibitor that has been approved recently for chronic plaque psoriasis (Roflumilast cream).

- Phototherapy: Ultraviolet radiation is locally immunosuppressive. Narrowband ultraviolet B radiation is the most commonly used phototherapy modality for Psoriasis. Side effects include burning and a slight potential for photocarcinogenesis. It can be combined with and application of crude coal tar or dithranol (Griffiths et al. 2021).

- Oral drugs available for moderate to severe psoriasis include methotrexate, apremilast, cyclosporin, fumarates and acetretin (Menter et al. 2011).

- Among these cyclosporin has a better efficacy rate than others (Gudjonsson and Elder 2019).

- Cyclosporin doses up to 5 mg/kg per day are used in adults. The side effects include hypertension, hypomagnesemia, hyperkalemia and hyperlipidemia. May not be suitable for long-term use due to irreversible nephrotoxicity. Therefore, should not be used for more than one year (Ellis et al. 1991)

- Methotrexate: Oral methotrexate 7.5–15 mg weekly is the usual adult dose. It is usually administered as single dose weekly. Complete blood count (CBC), basic metabolic panel (BMP), hepatic function panel baseline labs needs to be done prior to starting methotrexate. Thereafter, patients need to be monitored with regular CBC and hepatic function tests.

- Apremilast 30 mg orally twice daily in adults is also another feasible option in primary care. Depression, gastro intestinal disturbances and weight loss are the common side effects.

- Acetretin 25–50 mg per day orally is the usual adult dose.

- Biologics: These are often recombinant monoclonal antibodies or receptor fusion proteins and target specific inflammatory mediators. The biologics available to treat psoriasis in adults can be classified into 4 types: Anti-TNFα, Anti-IL17, Anti-IL-12p40 or IL-23p40, and Anti-IL-23p19 (Griffiths et al. 2021).

- Anti-TNFα agents in use for psoriasis include adalimumab, certolizumab pegol, etanercept and infliximab (Reich et al. 2005).

- Anti-IL-17 agents include secukinumab, ixekizumab and brodalumab (Griffiths et al. 2021).

- Anti-IL-23 agents include ustekinumab, that blocks the common p40 subunit of IL-12 and IL-23, and guselkumab, risankizumab and tildrakizumab. The latter three target the p19 subunit of IL-23.

- Biologics are highly effective. However, not all patients respond in the same manner. Some patients may not respond at all or, more commonly, have an initial response that is subsequently lost over a period of time (Griffiths et al. 2021).

3.1.2 Guttate Psoriasis

- Commonly seen in young adults.

- Guttate psoriasis is characterized by eruption of small papules or plaques (Fig. 3.2).

- Trunk and proximal extremities are common sites.

- A preceding episode of pharyngitis or tonsillitis occurs in about two thirds of patients and approximately half have elevated antistreptolysin O, anti-DNase B, or streptozyme titers (Quimby et al. 1980).

- Guttate psoriasis is often self-limited with spontaneous resolution in 6–12 weeks. About 40% of cases progress to chronic plaque psoriasis (Martin 1996).

- Anti-streptococcal antibiotics therapy is administered, if culture is positive. However, the role of antibiotics in the management of guttate psoriasis is unclear; tonsillectomy has shown some benefit in recurrent cases associated with tonsillitis (Dupire et al. 2019; Rachakonda et al. 2015).

Fig. 3.2 Guttate psoriasis

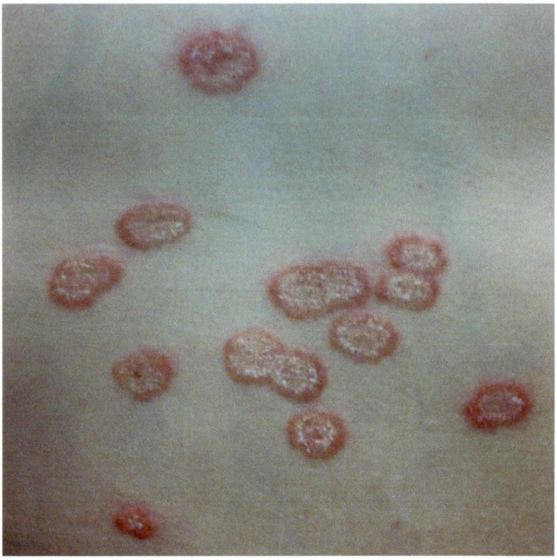

- **Treatment**: Treatment may not be needed in mild cases of guttate psoriasis but with extensive disease, broad band ultraviolet B (UVB) phototherapy is better than other phototherapy options (Saleh et al. 2023). It could be combined with topical therapy. Topical therapy is usually with ultra potent corticosteroids.

3.1.3 Variants of Psoriasis Based on the Site of Involvement

- **Inverse psoriasis or flexural psoriasis**: It is manifested as well demarcated, erythematous patches in the body folds. The surface is shiny, smooth and moist. The characteristic scaling that is associated with chronic plaque type is usually absent. The most common areas affected are the inguinal folds, followed by axillae, inframammary folds, perianal area, umbilicus and retroauricular areas (Micali et al. 2019).

- Other flexural areas such as antecubital and popliteal fossae and interdigital spaces can also be involved. Given that the flexural skin is generally thinner, first line of treatment is application of low to moderate potent topical steroids for short term (Micali et al. 2019) and calcineurin inhibitors and vitamin D analogues to be used for long term if needed.

- **Palmoplantar psoriasis**: Most commonly manifests as hyperkeratotic, fissured plaques on the palms and soles. Treatment is with ultrapotent topical steroids such as clobetasol propionate 0.05% ointment. Calcineurin inhibitors (Tacrolimus and pimecrolimus) and vitamin D analogues (Calcipotriene) can also be used if needed for long term.

– Please see Chap. 11, Upper extremity and Hands Figs. 11.12 and 11.13 for pictures of Palmoplantar psoriasis and also for more details on the clinical manifestations and management.

– **Sebopsoriasis** occurs in the scalp and seborrheic areas such as eyebrows, nasolabial folds, postauricular and presternal areas.

3.2 Lichen Planus (LP)

– Lichen planus is a chronic lichenoid inflammatory disorder of the skin, as well as mucosa and of the appendages (Solimani et al. 2021).

– The exact cause of lichen planus is unknown (Mangold and Pittelkow 2019).

– Clinically, there are three major subtypes: Cutaneous LP (CLP), Mucosal LP (MLP) and LP of the scalp, Lichen planopilaris (LPP) (Cleach and Chosidow 2012). These subtypes may occur in isolation or in combination.

– The cutaneous LP (CLP) lesions are well-marginated, flat topped, red-violet polygonal papules (Fig. 3.3). Papules coalesce into plaques.

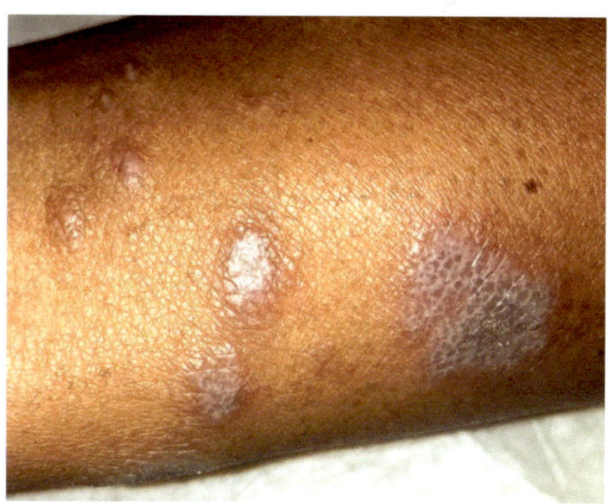

Fig. 3.3 Cutaneous Lichen planus

- Usually associated with intense itching.
- The distribution of the eruption is symmetrical with predilection for the flexural wrists, arms and legs.
- White, adherent reticulate scale can be noted in well-developed lesions—Wickham striae.
- Wickham striae are characteristic of lichen planus (Mangold and Pittelkow 2019).
- Oral involvement occurs in approximately 60–70% of patients, and in 20–30% of patients it could be the sole manifestation (Silverman et al. 1985; Mangold and Pittelkow 2019).
- The reticular form of oral lichen planus is the most common. Often it is asymptomatic. The most common site is the buccal mucosa; followed by the tongue and gingiva (Mangold and Pittelkow 2019).
- Genital involvement can also occur (Fig. 3.4). It can coexist with oral LP.
- Nail involvement occurs in about 10% of cutaneous lichen planus patients (Solimani et al. 2021).

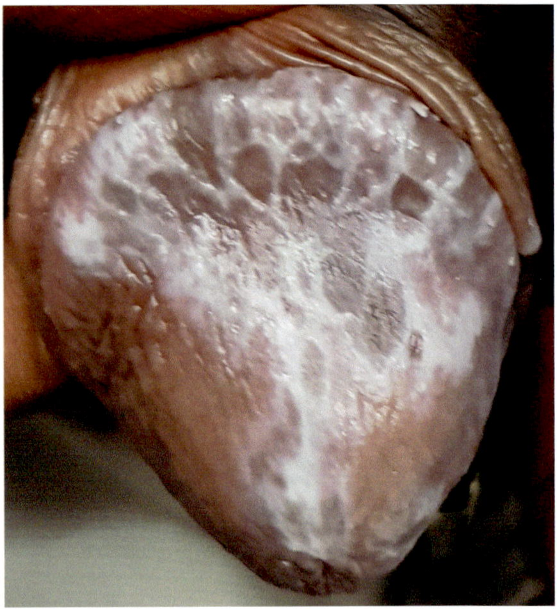

Fig. 3.4 Genital LP. *Courtesy* Dr. P.V. Krishna Rao, Dermatologist, India

- Both nail and mucosal LP can present in isolation or along with cutaneous LP.

- The most common findings of nail lichen planus are diffuse nail involvement with thinning, longitudinal ridging and distal nail splitting (onychoschizia) (Solimani et al. 2021).

- Pterygium or forward growth of the eponychia with adherence to the proximal nail plate is a classic finding in nail lichen planus involving the matrix.

- CLP like drug eruption can be caused by drugs. Anti-malarials, NSAIDs, thiazides, sulfonylurea, anti-tuberculous drugs, tumor necrosis factor (TNF) alfa drugs and gold are among them (Breathnach 2010; Gupta et al. 2015; Asarch et al. 2009).

- Most cutaneous lichen planus resolves within one to 2 years and may be associated with relapses (Solimani et al. 2021).

- Mucosal LP can have a chronic and relapsing course.

- Lichen planopilaris: Lichen plano pilaris (LPP) is a chronic, inflammatory disorder of the scalp manifested with red to purple papules and perifollicular erythema. This leads to destruction of hair follicles and eventually to non-reversible scarring alopecia of the scalp (Solimani et al. 2021).

3.2.1 Diagnosis

- The diagnosis of lichen planus is largely clinical. However, in cases with atypical or overlapping clinical features, a histopathologic diagnosis may be required.

3.2.2 Management

- CLP: Localized lesions can be treated with topical potent steroids like betamethasone dipropionate 0.05% ointment. Topical calcineurin inhibitors (Tacrolimus and pimecrolimus) can also be used as second line of drugs (Solimani et al. 2021).

- Generalized CLP can be treated with oral prednisone. Metronidazole, (Rasi et al. 2010) hydroxychloroquine, methotrexate, cyclosporine can also be used. So, also Narrowband UVB, PUVA (Psoralen plus Ultraviolet A) or Acitretin (Solimani et al. 2021).

- Mucosal LP: Oral LP: The initial topical treatment is with potent corticosteroids. They are usually used in an adhesive paste form. These are to be applied twice daily for about 1–2 months, and then tapered. Systemic corticosteroids can be used in short bursts in recalcitrant cases. Systemic methotrexate once weekly and oral cyclosporine can also be used (Lajevardi et al. 2016; Attwa et al. 2019).

- LPP: Topical application of potent steroids is the initial treatment of choice. Alternatively, topical calcineurin inhibitors can also be used. Simultaneous treatment with oral prednisone can be beneficial when the condition is more aggressive and rapidly progressing. Hydroxychloroquine or methotrexate can also be used (Jorge et al. 2018; Saber et al. 2017).

- Please note that there are some studies that showed association between LP and Hepatitis C Virus (HCV) infection. There is no universal recommendation for screening LP patients for HCV infection.

3.3 Pityriasis Rosea

- Pityriasis rosea is an acute, self-limited papulosquamous disorder.

- Children and young adults are commonly affected.

- Although exact etiology is not certain, human herpesvirus (HHV)-7 and HHV-6 have been implicated as the causative agents in some patients with pityriasis rosea (Canpolat Kirac et al. 2009).

- It has distinct clinical presentation.

- The initial presentation is usually in the form of an isolated oval plaque that has a colarette of fine scale just inside the periphery (Fig. 3.5). This plaque is called a herald patch or mother patch.

- Trunk is the common location of herald patch.

- Within few days, this is followed by an eruption of daughter patches that are smaller but similar in appearance. These occur on the trunk and proximal extremities, usually with their long axis along the lines of cleavage—A christmas tree pattern (Villalon-Gomez 2018).

- Sometimes herald patch may be absent and patient may only manifest with lesions that are similar to daughter patches.

- Self-limiting in about 6–8 weeks.

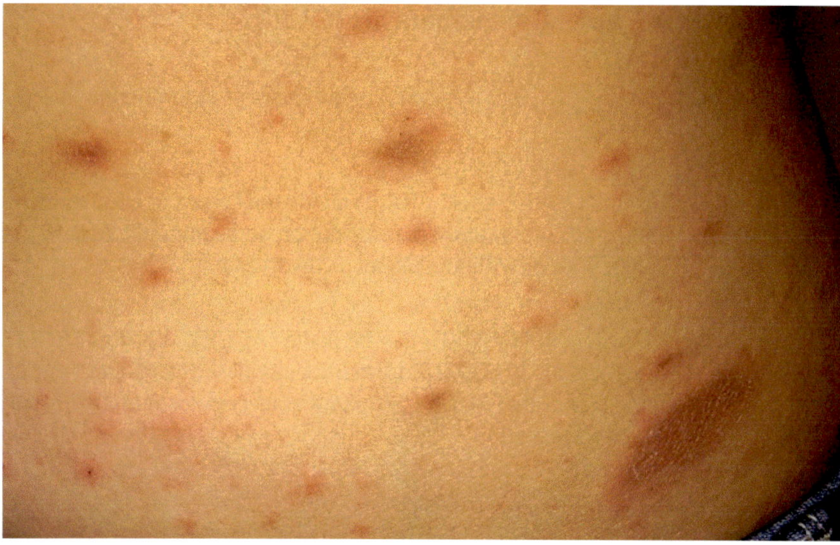

Fig. 3.5 Pityriasis rosea (Herald patch seen towards the right side of the picture)

3.3.1 Diagnosis

- Diagnosis is made clinically. In classical presentations, diagnosis is usually straightforward. When the herald patch is not present or when there are clinical variants, the diagnosis can be challenging. Sometimes, herald patch can be confused with tinea corporis. Tinea corporis is itchy with central clearing and raised borders. Please see the chapter on cutaneous infections for more details about the presentation of tinea corporis.

3.3.2 Management

- Supportive. Reassurance and symptomatic treatment with emollients and antihistamine is adequate in most cases as the disease is self-limiting. Active intervention in the form of oral acyclovir, macrolides (more so erythromycin) and ultraviolet therapy in severe or recurrent cases (or in pregnant women) may be considered. If active intervention is needed, there is evidence to support the use of oral acyclovir to shorten the duration of illness (Leung et al. 2020).

- Pitfalls: Secondary syphilis is a deadly trap. Secondary syphilis could also present with scaly plaques with colarette of scaling. But, it can involve palms and soles and ulceration in the oral cavity can also occur. There could be constitutional symptoms and generalized lymphadenopathy can also be noted. When in doubt, serological testing needs to be done to rule out syphilis.

3.4 Cutaneous Lupus Erythematosus (CLE)

- Lupus erythematosus (LE) is a chronic, inflammatory, autoimmune disease (Wenzel 2019).

- CLE and systemic lupus erythematosus (SLE) are distinct types of LE. Dermatological components of LE are described under the broad heading CLE. SLE has systemic involvement with or without cutaneous involvement.

- Cutaneous lupus erythematosus (CLE) can be acute (ACLE), subacute (SCLE) and chronic (CLE) (Lu et al. 2021). CLE is traditionally described under connective tissue disorders. Given that SCLE can manifest as papulosqumous lesions, CLE is described in this chapter.

3.4.1 Acute Cutaneous LE

- ACLE is often associated with SLE (Fabbri et al. 2003).

- It often manifests as photosensitive rash in the malar region of the face-butterfly rash. The rash is erythematous and transient triggered by sunlight.

- Sometimes ACLE can also manifest as a more extensive form consisting of maculopapular lesions in a photosensitive distribution involving upper extremities and other sun exposed parts of the body (Vale and Garcia 2023).

- Mucosal involvement in the form or erosions or ulcers is common (Vale and Garcia 2023).

3.4.2 Subacute Cutaneous LE

- SCLE manifests as small, erythematous, slightly scaly papules that transform into either psoriasiform plaques or polycyclic annular plaques (Vale and Garcia 2023)

- The lesions are often photodistributed and thus common sites include the shoulders, extensors of forearms (Figs. 3.6 and 3.7), V of the chest and upper part of the back of the trunk. Face is often spared. Scarring usually does not occur.

- Photosensitivity is present.

- Several classes of drugs have been implicated in SCLE. Examples include antihypertensive drugs, proton pump inhibitors, lipid lowering drugs, anti-fungal

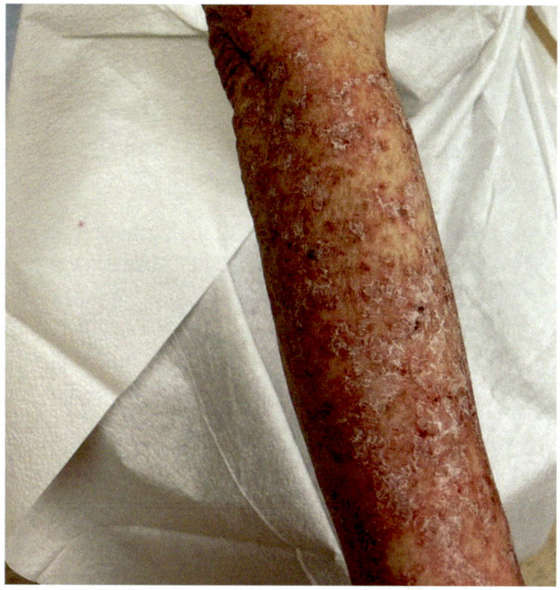

Fig. 3.6 Subacute cutaneous lupus erythematosus

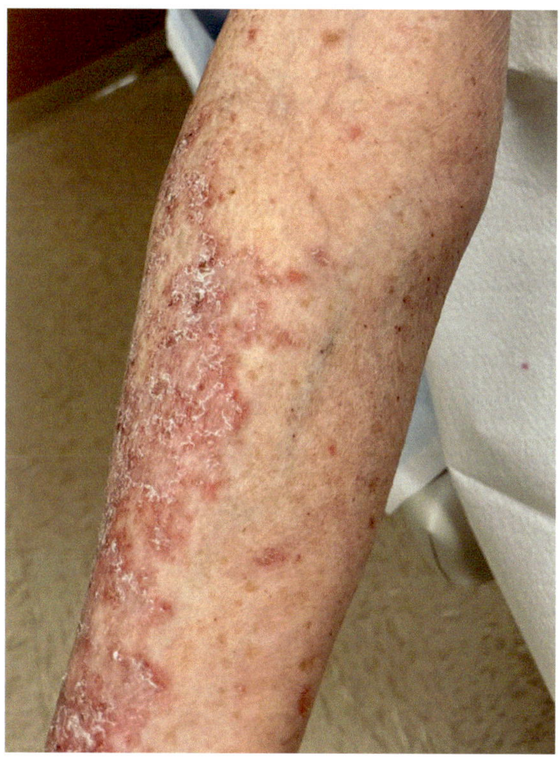

Fig. 3.7 Subacute cutaneous lupus erythematosus. Inner aspect of the extremity is spared

agents and TNF-alpha inhibitors. Withdrawal of culprit drugs often can lead to improvement of drug induced SCLE (Marzano et al. 2011)

- More than 80% of patients with SCLE have anti-Ro/SSA antibodies. (Lin et al. 2007; Marzano et al. 2011).

- Approximately 50% of patients with SCLE meet the American College of Rheumatology (ACR)'s revised criteria for the classification of SLE (Cohen and Crosby 1994).

3.4.3 Chronic Cutaneous LE

- Discoid Lupus Erythematosus (DLE) is the most predominant form of CLE.

- DLE can be either localized or generalized. It is said to be localized if it involves only above the neck. The localized form is more common.

- Classic or localized DLE lesions are characterized by erythematous, scaly plaques with dyspigmentation. Lesions are hyperpigmented peripherally. Hypopigmentation and depigmentation can be present in the center. Also associated with atrophy and follicular keratotic plugging (Okon and Werth 2013) (Fig. 3.8).

- Erythema and scaling indicate active disease.

- Head and neck are commonly involved.

- If conchal bowl is involved, it provides a diagnostic clue (Pearson 2022) (Fig. 3.9).

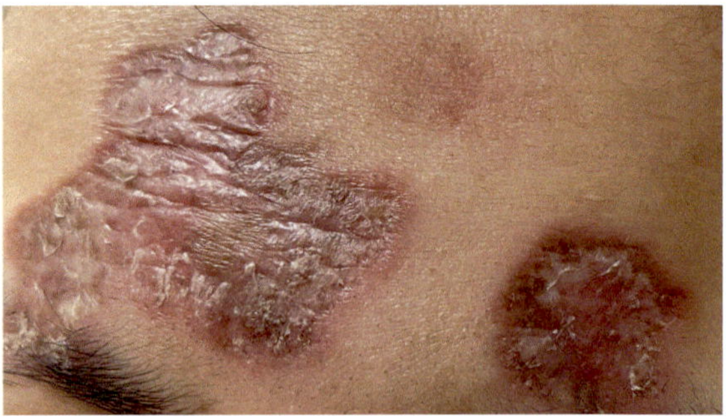

Fig. 3.8 Discoid lupus erythematosus

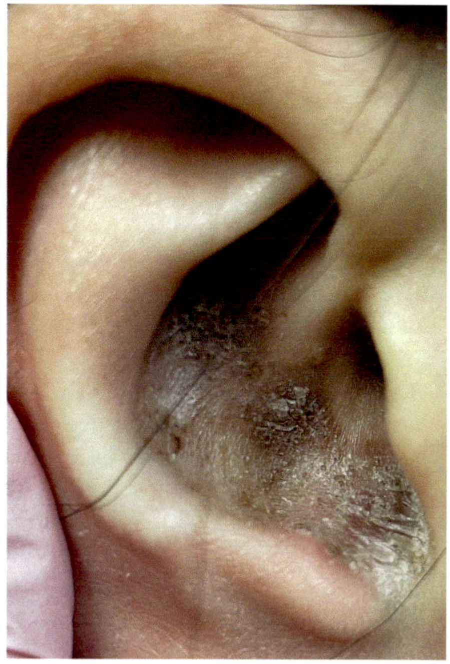

Fig. 3.9 Discoid lupus erythematosus involving conchal bowl

- DLE leads to scarring alopecia in hair-bearing areas. Please see Fig. 3.5 in Chap. 8 'Scalp' for a picture of DLE on scalp.

- Generalized DLE tends to typically involve hands and extensors of forearms (Walling and Sontheimer 2009).

- About 5–10% of DLE patients will progress to SLE; patients with generalized DLE have greater risk to progress to SLE (Crowson and Magro 2001; Chong et al. 2011; Vera-Recabarren et al. 2009; Okon and Werth 2013).

- Serologically, when compared to other forms of CLE, patients with DLE are less likely to be positive for ANA, dsDNA and Ro/SSA antibodies (McCauliffe 2001).

3.4.4 *Diagnosis of CLE*

- Histopathology and serology along with typical clinical presentation can confirm the diagnosis. It is essential that in all types of CLE, SLE be ruled out.

3.4.5 *Management of CLE*

- Photoprotection and smoking cessation is recommended in all CLE patients. Treatment includes topical potent corticosteroids, topical calcineurin inhibitors, and/or systemic glucocorticoids depending on the extent of involvement and subset of disease.

- It is essential that in all types of CLE, SLE be ruled out. Given the chronicity of CLE and its need for long-term monitoring, it is recommended that every patient of CLE be referred to a dermatologist for long term management.

- Topical potent corticosteroids such as betamethasone dipropionate 0.05% ointment are recommended as first-line treatment for a short term (up to several weeks) in all CLE lesions. The scalp lesions may require prolonged use of topical corticosteroids. Intralesional injection of corticosteroids for localized, refractory DLE is suggested (Lu et al. 2021).

- Calcineurin inhibitors are recommended as an alternative first-line option for topical treatment of DLE (Kuhn et al. 2011; Lu et al. 2021).

- Anti-malarials, especially hydroxychloroquine (HCQ), is recommended as first-line systemic treatment in all CLE patients with widespread or severe skin lesions (McCauliffe 2001).

- The recommended daily dose of HCQ is $\leq$ 5 mg/kg real body weight. In those who do not have any risk factors for retinopathy, an ophthalmological examination is recommended at baseline and annually after 5 years of starting treatment with HCQ. However, in those with already risk factors for retinopathy, annual opthalmological screening is recommended upon starting HCQ (Lu et al. 2021).

- In addition to HCQ, systemic corticosteroids are recommended as first-line treatment in patients with severe or widespread active CLE lesions. Gradual tapering and final discontinuation of systemic corticosteroids is recommended after CLE becomes under control. Continuation of treatment with anti-malarials or other corticosteroids-sparing agents is recommended during the tapering and after discontinuation of systemic corticosteroids (Lu et al. 2021).

3.5 Pityriasis Versicolor (Tinea Versicolor)

- It is a type of superficial fungal infection. Given that it has some fine scaling, sometimes it can come under the differential diagnosis of papulosquamous disorders.

- It is caused mainly by yeast. Malasazzia furfur and Malasazzia globosa are the common species (Saizan and Elbuluk 2022).

- Manifests as well demarcated macules or patches that are either pink or hyperpigmented (Fig. 3.10) or hypo pigmented (on dark skin).

- There is a fine scaling.

- Besides the trunk, neck and upper extremities can also be involved (Brandi et al. 2019).

- Asymptomatic.

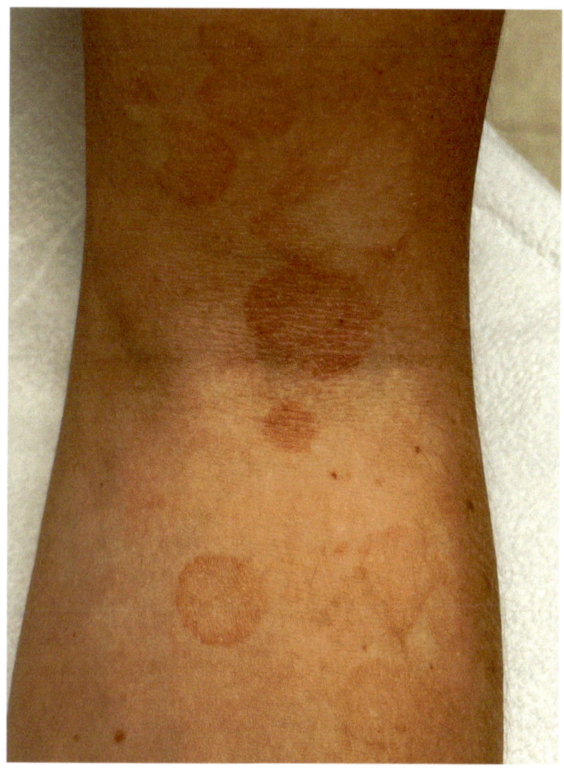

Fig. 3.10 Pityriasis versicolor

3.5.1 *Diagnosis*

- Clinical findings confirmed with positive potassium hydroxide (KOH) preparation findings.

- Microscopic examination of scales prepared with KOH shows filamentous hyphae and globose forms of yeast, a 'spaghetti and meatballs' appearance (Saizan and Elbuluk 2022).

- Wood's lamp and skin biopsy also help, with the former showing copper-orange or yellowish-white fluorescence of scales (Ponka and Baddar 2012).

3.5.2 *Management*

- Topical selenium sulfide (2.5%) lotion or shampoo, or ketoconazole shampoo or azole creams (ketoconazole, econazole, micronazole, or clotrimazole) or terbinafine 1% solution.

- Systemic therapy in adults: Fluconazole and itraconazole are options (Karray et al. 2022).

- Please note the dyspigmentation can persist for months even after infection is cleared.

3.6 Seborrheic Dermatitis

- Seborrheic dermatitis (Fig. 3.11) is a type of endogenous eczema that is manifested with greasy looking scales involving seborrheic areas such as scalp, eyebrows, glabella, nasolabial folds, tip of the chin, front of the chest and pubic area. Please see Chap. 5 'Eczema' for clinical features, diagnosis and management of Seborrheic dermatitis.

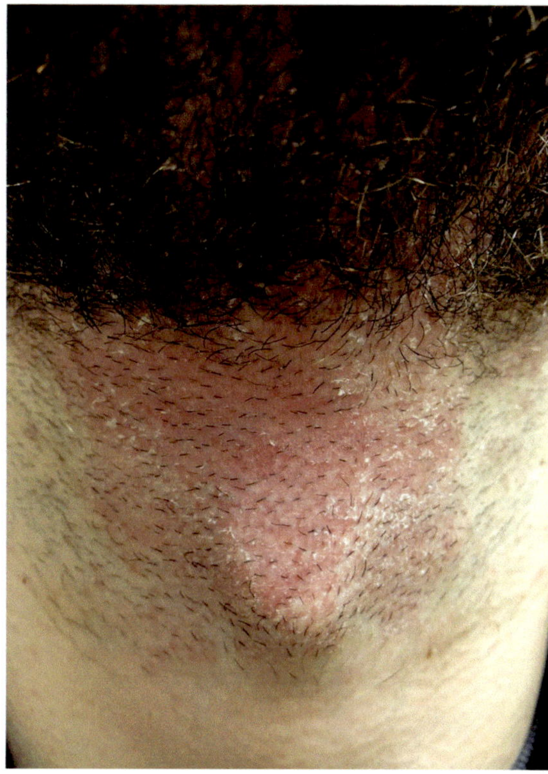

Fig. 3.11 Seborrheic Dermatitis

3.7 Tinea Corporis

– It is a superficial fungal infection that is caused by dermatophytes. The lesions of tinea corporis show central clearing with raised borders. It can have some fine scaling and thus sometimes comes in the differential diagnosis of papulosqumous disorders such as pityriasis rosea. Please see Chap. 6 'Common Cutaneous Infections' for clinical features, diagnosis and management of tinea corporis.

As a summary, Table 3.1 shows salient features of the scaly disorders discussed above.

Table 3.1 A summary of salient features of the papulosquamous disorders & other conditions that can mimic them

Skin disorder	Salient clinical features
Psoriasis	Minimal or no itching, distribution: extensors, silvery adherent scales Nail changes (please see the text)
Lichen planus	Intense itching Distribution: flexors, violate, flat topped, polygonal papules/plaques Oral mucosa can be involved Nail changes (please see the text)
Pityriais rosea	Minimal or no itching H/O Herald patch with daughter patches is usually present Distribution: commonly involves trunk Peripheral colarette of scaling noted
Tinea corporis	Itching present. Central clearing and borders are raised. Fine scaling present
Seborrheic dermatitis	Greasy looking scales present in seborrheic areas such as scalp, eyebrows, glabella, nasolabial folds, tip of the chin, front of chest and pubic area
Subacute LE	Minimal or no itching. Distribution: sun exposed parts like outer aspects of upper extremities, V area of the chest and upper back
Pityriasis versicolor	Well-demarcated macules or patches that are either pink or hyperpigmented or hypopigmented (on dark skin). Fine scaling. Asymptomatic. Trunk and upper extremities are commonly involved

Bibliography

Asarch A, Gottlieb AB, Lee J, Masterpol KS, Scheinman PL, Stadecker MJ, et al. Lichen planus–like eruptions: an emerging side effect of tumor necrosis factor-α antagonists. J Am Acad Dermatol. 2009;61(1):104–11.

Attwa EM, Elkot RA, Abdelshafey AS, Hafez AR. Subcutaneous methotrexate versus oral form for the treatment and prophylaxis of chronic plaque psoriasis. Dermatol Therapy. 2019;32(5).

Brandi N, Starace M, Alessandrini A, Piraccini BM. Tinea versicolor of the neck as side effect of topical steroids for alopecia areata. J Dermatol Treat. 2019;30(8):757–9.

Breathnach S. Drug reactions. In: Burns T, Breathnach S, Cox N, Griffiths C, editors. Rook's textbook of dermatology, vol 4. 8th ed. Oxford: Blackwell Science; 2010. p. 73.1, 177.

Canpolat Kirac B, Adisen E, Bozdayi G, Yucel A, Fidan I, Aksakal N, et al. The role of human herpesvirus 6, human herpesvirus 7, Epstein-Barr virus and cytomegalovirus in the aetiology of pityriasis rosea. J Euro Acad Dermatol Venereol JEADV. 2009;23(1):16–21. Available from https://pubmed.ncbi.nlm.nih.gov/18713231/.

Chong BF, Song J, Olsen NJ. Determining risk factors for developing systemic lupus erythematosus in patients with discoid lupus erythematosus. Br J Dermatol. 2011;166(1):29–35.

Cohen MR, Crosby D. Systemic disease in subacute cutaneous lupus erythematosus: a controlled comparison with systemic lupus erythematosus. PubMed. 1994;21(9):1665–9.

Crowson AN, Magro C. The cutaneous pathology of lupus erythematosus: a review. J Cutan Pathol. 2001;28(1):1–23.

do Vale ECS, Garcia LC. Cutaneous lupus erythematosus: a review of etiopathogenic, clinical, diagnostic and therapeutic aspects. Anais Brasileiros de Dermatologia. 2023.

Dupire G, Droitcourt C, Hughes C, Le Cleach L. Antistreptococcal interventions for guttate and chronic plaque psoriasis. Cochrane Database Syst Rev. 2019.

Ellis CN, Fradin MS, Messana JM, Brown MD, Siegel MT, Hartley AH, et al. Cyclosporine for plaque-type psoriasis. N Engl J Med. 1991;324(5):277–84.

Fabbri P, Cardinali C, Giomi B, Caproni M. Cutaneous lupus erythematosus: diagnosis and management. Am J Clin Dermat. 2003;4(7):449–65.

Griffiths CEM, Armstrong AW, Gudjonsson JE, Barker JNWN. Psoriasis. Lancet. 2021;397(10281):1301–15.

Gudjonsson JE, Karason A, Hjaltey Runarsdottir E, Antonsdottir AA, Hauksson VB, Jónsson HH, et al. Distinct clinical differences between HLA-Cw*0602 positive and negative psoriasis patients—an analysis of 1019 HLA-C- and HLA-B-typed patients. J Investig Dermatol. 2006;126(4):740–5.

Gudjonsson JE, Elder JT. Psoriasis. In: Kang S, Amagai M, Bruckner AL, Enk AH, Margolis DJ, McMichael AJ, Orringer JS, editors. Fitzpatrick's Dermatology, 9e. McGraw-Hill Education; 2019.

Gupta M, Gupta H, Gupta A. Tenofovir induced lichenoid drug eruption. Avicenna J Med. 2015;5(3):95.

Jorge AM, Melles RB, Zhang Y, Lu N, Rai SK, Young LH, et al. Hydroxychloroquine prescription trends and predictors for excess dosing per recent ophthalmology guidelines. Arthritis Res Ther. 2018;20(1).

Karray M, McKinney WP. Tinea versicolor. 2022 Aug 8. In: StatPearls. Treasure Island: StatPearls Publishing; 2024. PMID: 29494106.

Kuhn A, Gensch K, Haust M, Schneider SW, Bonsmann G, Gaebelein-Wissing N, et al. Efficacy of tacrolimus 0.1% ointment in cutaneous lupus erythematosus: a multicenter, randomized, double-blind, vehicle-controlled trial. J Am Acad Dermatol. 2011;65(1):54–64.e2.

Lajevardi V, Ghodsi SZ, Hallaji Z, Shafiei Z, Aghazadeh N, Akbari Z. Treatment of erosive oral lichen planus with methotrexate. JDDG J der Deutschen Dermatologischen Gesellschaft. 2016;14(3):286–93.

Le Cleach L, Chosidow O. Lichen planus. N Engl J Med. 2012;366(8):723–32.

Leung AKC, Lam JM, Leong KF, Hon KL. Pityriasis rosea: an updated review. Curr Pediatric Rev. 2020. Available from https://pubmed.ncbi.nlm.nih.gov/32964824/.

Lin J, Dutz JP, Sontheimer RD, Werth VP. Pathophysiology of cutaneous lupus erythematosus. 2007;33(1–2):85–106.

Lu Q, Long H, Chow S, Hidayat S, Danarti R, Listiawan Y, et al. Guideline for the diagnosis, treatment and long-term management of cutaneous lupus erythematosus. 2021;123:102707–7.

Mangold AR, Pittelkow MR. Lichen planus. In: Kang S, Amagai M, Bruckner AL, Enk AH, Margolis DJ, McMichael AJ, Orringer JS, editors. Fitzpatrick's Dermatology, 9e. McGraw-Hill Education; 2019.

Martin BA. How great is the risk of further psoriasis following a single episode of acute guttate psoriasis? Arch Dermatol. 1996;132(6):717.

Marzano AV, Lazzari R, Polloni I, Crosti C, Fabbri P, Cugno M. Drug-induced subacute cutaneous lupus erythematosus: evidence for differences from its idiopathic counterpart. Br J Dermatol. 2011;165(2):335–41.

McCauliffe DP. Cutaneous lupus erythematosus. Semin Cutan Med Surg. 2001;20(1):14–26.

Menter A, Korman NJ, Elmets CA, Feldman SR, Gelfand JM, Gordon KB, et al. Guidelines of care for the management of psoriasis and psoriatic arthritis. J Am Acad Dermatol. 2011;65(1):137–74.

Micali G, Verzì AE, Giuffrida G, Panebianco E, Musumeci ML, Lacarrubba F. Inverse psoriasis: from diagnosis to current treatment options. Clin Cosmetic Investigational Dermatol. 2019;12(12):953–9. Available from https://www.ncbi.nlm.nih.gov/pmc/articles/PMC6997231/.

Okon LG, Werth VP. Cutaneous lupus erythematosus: diagnosis and treatment. Best Pract Res Clin Rheumatol. 2013;27(3):391–404.

Pearson DR. Skin signs of systemic disease. In: Soutor C, Hordinsky MK, editors. Clinical dermatology: diagnosis and management of common disorders, 2e. McGraw-Hill Education; 2022.

Ponka D, Baddar F. Wood lamp examination. Canadian Family Physician. 2012;58(9):976. Available from https://www.ncbi.nlm.nih.gov/pmc/articles/PMC3440273/.

Quimby S, Markowitz H, Winkelmann R. Antideoxyribonuclease B titers in psoriasis. Acta Derm Venereol. 1980;60(6):485–90.

Rachakonda TD, Dhillon JS, Florek AG, Armstrong AW. Effect of tonsillectomy on psoriasis: a systematic review. J Am Acad Dermatol. 2015;72(2):261–75.

Rasi A, Behzadi AH, Davoudi S, Rafizadeh P, Honarbakhsh Y, Mehran M et al. Efficacy of oral metronidazole in treatment of cutaneous and mucosal lichen planus. PubMed. 2010;9(10):1186–90.

Reich K, Nestle FO, Papp K, Ortonne JP, Evans R, Guzzo C, et al. Infliximab induction and maintenance therapy for moderate-to-severe psoriasis: a phase III, multicentre, double-blind trial. Lancet. 2005;366(9494):1367–74. Available from https://www.ncbi.nlm.nih.gov/pubmed/16226614.

Roflumilast cream, for topical use. US Food and Drug Administration (FDA) approved product information. Revised July 2022. US Food and Drug Administration. https://www.accessdata.fda.gov/drugsatfda_docs/label/2022/215985s000lbl.pdf.

Saber M, Naeini F, Asilian A, Hosseini S. Clinical efficacy and safety of methotrexate versus hydroxychloroquine in preventing lichen planopilaris progress: a randomized clinical trial. Int J Prev Med. 2017;8(1):37.

Saizan AL, Elbuluk N. Pigmentary disorders. In: Soutor C, Hordinsky MK, editors. Clinical dermatology: diagnosis and management of common disorders, 2e. McGraw-Hill Education; 2022.

Saleh D, Tanner LS. Guttate Psoriasis. 2023 Jul 31. In: StatPearls. Treasure Island: StatPearls Publishing; 2024. PMID: 29494104.

Silverman S, Gorsky M, Lozada-Nur F. A prospective follow-up study of 570 patients with oral lichen planus: persistence, remission, and malignant association. Oral Surg Oral Med Oral Pathol. 1985;60(1):30–4.

Solimani F, Forchhammer S, Schloegl A, Ghoreschi K, Meier K. Lichen planus—a clinical guide. JDDG J der Deutschen Dermatologischen Gesellschaft. 2021;19(6):864–82.

Vera-Recabarren MA, García-Carrasco M, Ramos-Casals M, Herrero C. Comparative analysis of subacute cutaneous lupus erythematosus and chronic cutaneous lupus erythematosus: clinical and immunological study of 270 patients. Br J Dermatol. 2009;162(1):91–101.

Villalon-Gomez JM. Pityriasis rosea: diagnosis and treatment. Am Fam Physician. 2018;97(1):38–44.

Walling HW, Sontheimer RD. Cutaneous lupus erythematosus. Am J Clin Dermatol. 2009;10(6):365–81.

Wenzel J. Cutaneous lupus erythematosus: new insights into pathogenesis and therapeutic strategies. Nat. Rev. Rheumatol. 2019;15(9):519–32. Available from https://www.nature.com/articles/s41584-019-0272-0.

Wilson FC, Icen M, Crowson CS, McEvoy MT, Gabriel SE, Kremers HM. Incidence and clinical predictors of psoriatic arthritis in patients with psoriasis: a population-based study. Arthritis Rheumatism. 2009;61(2):233–9. Available from https://doi.org/10.1002/art.24172.

Chapter 4
Vesiculo Bullous Lesions (Blistering Rashes)

Abstract Vesiculo bullous lesions are commonly encountered in primary care. The notable conditions that present with blisters are the following. This chapter provides clinical tips regarding the diagnosis and management of these conditions.

Contact dermatitis
Insect bites
Herpes simplex
Herpes zoster
Bullous impetigo
Hand foot mouth disease
Bullous pemphigoid
Pemphigus vulgaris.

Keywords Bullous pemphigoid · Pemphigus vulgaris · Blisters · Vesicular rash · Hand foot mouth disease · Insect bites · Herpes simplex · Herpes zoster

4.1 Contact Dermatitis

4.1.1 Diagnostic Tips

- History of exposure to an offending agent such as poison ivy is usually given but not always.
- Also, patient can sometimes give you prior history of having similar presentation upon exposure to an offending agent such as poison ivy.
- Can be localized or generalized.

D. K. Yellumahanthi, *Manual of Primary Care Dermatology*,
https://doi.org/10.1007/978-3-031-68406-7_4

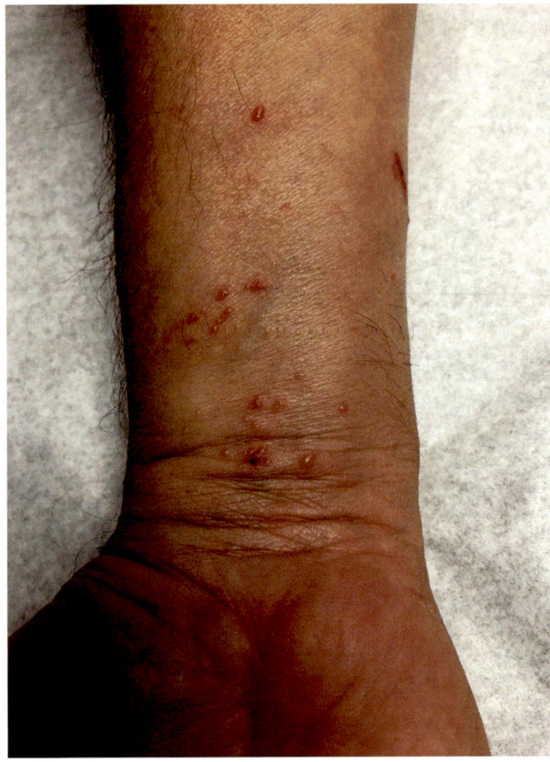

Fig. 4.1 Contact dermatitis to poison ivy

- Blisters can be noticed in acute stages. Presence of blisters in a linear fashion suggesting contact with an extraneous source along that path, is often present. Please see a linear lesion near the ulnar border of Fig. 4.1.

4.1.2 Management

- Identifying and eliminating the offending agent is the initial step.

- Depending on the body area, appropriate topical steroids can be given: For instance, on the face, desonide 0.05% cream, on the body other than face, depending on the severity, either hydrocortisone valerate 0.2% ointment or betamethasone dipropionate 0.05% ointment.

- Oral prednisone for a short duration can be given if the inflammation is extensive.

- Please see Chap. 5 'Eczema' for more details on the clinical manifestations, diagnosis and management of contact dermatitis.

4.2 Insect Bites

- Can be localized or generalized.
- History of exposure to insects may or may not always be elicited.
- The lesions are usually painful to some degree than mere itching.

4.2.1 Management

- In localized cases, topical antibiotics to prevent secondary infection and oral antihistamines are usually all that is needed. In more extensive cases, oral antibiotics to prevent secondary infection and oral steroids may have to be added as appropriate.

4.3 Herpes Simplex

- Caused by Herpes Simplex Virus (HSV) 1 and 2. HSV 1, usually presents as groups of blisters around the corners of the mouth and HSV 2 on the genitalia. Primary HSV1 can sometimes be severe leading to Herpetic gingivostomatitis.
- Please keep in mind, inoculated herpes can occur at any site on the body. Therefore, if grouped vesicles are present locally anywhere on the body, think of the possibility of herpes.
- Usually associated with pain or tingling sensation.

4.3.1 Management

- There are various regimens that includes either acyclovir or famciclovir or valacyclovir. For primary herpetic gingivitis, acyclovir could be a better option. If there are too frequent flare ups, suppressive therapy with antivirals can be initiated.
- Please see Chap. 6 'Common cutaneous infections' for more details on clinical manifestations, diagnosis and management of herpes simplex.

4.4 Herpes Zoster

- Blistering lesions occur along the dermatome. Therefore, seen in a ribbon shape or segmentally. The lesions are only on one side of the body and never cross the midline.

- Pain often precedes the rash by 2–3 days. But, can be longer sometimes.

- Rarely, herpes zoster could manifest only as pain along a dermatome without any skin lesions.

- Post herpetic neuralgia (PHN) is the dreaded complication. If significant pain persists beyond 90 days after the onset of the rash, it is termed as PHN.

4.4.1 Management

- Starting antivirals within 72 hours after the onset of rash, helps in reducing the intensity of acute symptoms of zoster. It is not clear exactly if antivirals also will benefit in reducing the chances of developing PHN. The following are the various regimens of antivirals used in adults:

  Valacylovir 1000 mg orally three times daily for 7 days.
  Famciclovir 500 mg orally three times daily for 7 days and
  Acyclovir 800 mg orally five times daily for seven days (Preferred regimen among pregnant women).

- The acute pain of zoster if not better with oral antivirals, Non Steroid Anti Inflammatory Drugs (NSAIDs) and opioids can help. If still not better gabapentin or pregabalin or a low dose of amitriptyline at bedtime can be tried.

- If PHN ensues, it is better to refer the patient to a dermatologist.

- Please see Chap. 6 'Common cutaneous infections' for more details on clinical manifestations, diagnosis and management of herpes zoster.

4.5 Bullous Impetigo

- More common in children.
- Tends to be more often localized.
- Flaccid bullae are seen.
- Please see Chap. 6 'Common cutaneous infections' for more details on clinical manifestations, diagnosis and management of bullous impetigo.

4.6 Hand Foot Mouth Disease

- Hand foot mouth disease is a viral exanthem caused by enteroviruses including coxsackievirus A16 and enterovirus 71 (Kimmis et al. 2018).
- Common in children in Summer and Fall.
- Associated with a brief non-specific prodrome consisting of low grade fever for 1–2 days, malaise and upper respiratory symptoms or abdominal pain.
- In addition to palms and soles, blisters can be present on the arms, buttocks and legs. An area of redness can be present at the base of some blisters (Hand Foot et al. 2019).
- Erosions in the mouth are also usually present.
- Diagnosis is made clinically.

4.6.1 Management

- Self-resolving without significant sequelae in the majority of cases.
- Treatment is supportive.

4.7 Bullous Pemphigoid (BP)

- Bullous pemphigoid (BP) often begins with pruritus and urticated and erythematous lesions. Subsequently, large tense blisters develop on both normal and erythematous skin. Blisters and erosions could also be present on the mucosa (Bullous pemphigoid)

- It is uncommon and mainly occurs in the elderly.

- Etiology: BP is an autoimmune disease and is characterized by IgG autoantibodies to hemidesmosome-associated proteins within the adhesion complex.

- The two major bullous antigens are BP230 and BP180, which are associated with hemidesmosomes (Pemphigoid et al. 2018).

- Drugs that can cause BP include Furosemide, penicillins, penicillamine, non-steroidal anti-inflammatory drugs, TNF alfa inhibitor drugs (Ruocco and Sacerdoti 1991; Béné et al. 2016).

4.7.1 *Clinical Features*

- It starts with itching and a non-specific rash on the limbs and trunk that may be either urticaria-like or occasionally eczematous.

- The urticarial prodrome usually lasts 1–3 weeks before blisters occur. (Bullous pemphigoid)

- Blisters may arise either on the erythematous area or on the normal skin.

- Blisters are tense and dome shaped (Fig. 4.2), could be of many centimeters in size.

- It mainly involves flexures of limbs and on the central abdomen.

- Mucosal involvement is uncommon occurring in about 10–30% of the patients with oral, esophageal and genital lesions (Pemphigoid et al. 2018) and when it does occur, it tends to be not clinically significant.

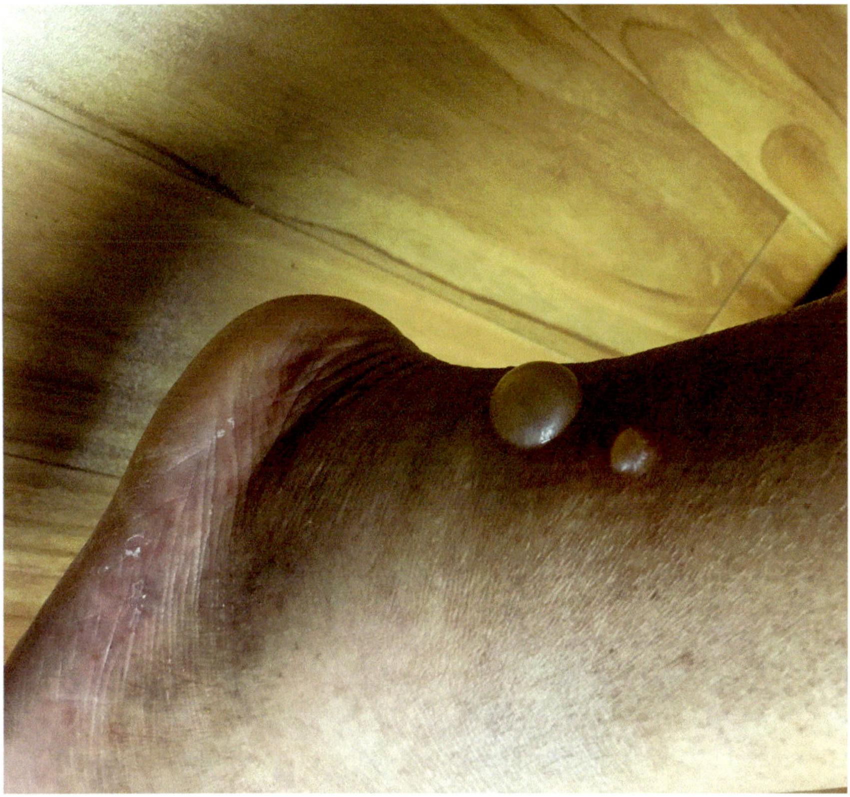

Fig. 4.2 Bulllous pemphigoid

4.7.2 Diagnosis

- Blood tests**:** In bullous pemphigoid, circulating pemphigoid antibodies can be quantified using techniques such as ELISA (Enzyme-linked immune sorbant assay) indirect immunofluorescence. The titers of autoantibody have been shown to correlate with disease activity (Schmidt et al. 2000).

- Skin biopsy: Blister is subepidermal and contains eosinophils, neutrophils and fibrin. It also has dermal inflammatory infiltrate (Lamberts et al. 2018).

- Direct immunofluorescence (DIF): DIF shows linear deposition of IgG and/or C3 to BP180 and BP230 along the basement membrane. Please note, perilesional skin is used for taking the sample for DIF.

4.7.3 *Management*

- If BP is generalized, it is better to refer to a dermatologist. Topical ultra (Super) potent steroids such as clobetasol propionate 0.05% ointment and systemic steroids are the first-line treatments (Pemphigoid et al. 2018) that can be given while waiting on seeing the dermatologist. Among adult patients,
- Azathioprine can also be used.
- Methotrexate, Dapsone can be tried.
- Doxycycline can be used as an adjuvant therapy. Doxycycline 200 mg per day for 6 weeks has been as efficacious as prednisolone 0.5 mg/kg/day (Williams et al. 2017).
- Rituximab, omalizumab have emerged as alternative treatment and are among the second line treatment (Pemphigoid et al. 2018).

4.7.4 *Prognosis*

- Untreated BP runs a chronic, self-limiting course over a period of several months to years.
- BP patients have around six times higher mortality than when compared to their counterparts who are healthy and age matched (Joly et al. 2012).

4.8 Pemphigus Vulgaris (PV)

- Pemphigus vulgaris is an uncommon immunobullous condition that is characterized by the formation of blisters and erosions on the skin. Mucosal involvement, more so of the mouth is also very common.
- In pemphigus, the blister formation is within the epidermis.

4.8.1 *Etiology*

- Pemphigus vulgaris is an immunobullous condition.

- Pemphigus vulgaris antigen, also known as desmoglein-3, is the desmosomal cadherin involved in mediating intercellular adhesion in the epidermis.

- IgG autoantibodies are produced against the PV antigen that results in the keratinocytes separation from each other, and are replaced by fluid, the blister (Pemphigus vulgaris and pemphigus vegetans)

4.8.2 Clinical Features

- Mucosal involvement occurs in about 90% of all patients (Malik et al. 2021) with oral lesions in 50–70% of the patients.

- These could precede skin lesions by months or be the only manifestation of the disease. Blisters are rarely seen. Painful erosions mainly involving the buccal mucosa, lips and palate are common.

- Cutaneous lesions are more common on the scalp, face, axillae, and groins. Flaccid blisters with clear fluid arise on normal skin or an erythematous base.

- Blisters as they are within the epidermis, are fragile and usually rupture, producing painful erosions. Lesions heal without scarring.

- Firm sliding pressure with a finger will separate normal-looking epidermis from dermis, producing an erosion—Nikolsky sign.

4.8.3 Diagnosis

- Blood tests: Pemphigus Vulgaris antibodies are detected in over 80% of cases. (Pemphigus vulgaris and pemphigus vegetans)

- Skin biopsy: Histolopathological examination shows suprabasilar acantholysis. There is retention of basal keratinocytes along the basement membrane (Malik et al. 2021).

- DIF shows IgG deposition on the surface of keratinocytes all through the epidermis, in and around lesions.

4.8.4 Management

- As we discussed with BP, PV also requires referral to a dermatologist. Systemic corticosteroids are first line of treatment. Often oral prednisone is the common agent used. (Melchionda and Harman 2019).

- Azathioprine and mycophenolate mofetil can be used as corticosteroid-sparing adjuvant therapies (Gregoriou et al. 2015; Joly et al. 2017).

- Rituximab, the chimeric anti-CD20 monoclonal antibody can be used for refractory disease or at the disease onset as well (Cholera and Chainani-Wu 2016; Boulard et al. 2016).

- Prednisone and azathioprine may be more effective than either of them separately.

- Dapsone can also be used an adjuvant therapy (Primary Care Dermatology Society).

- Cyclophosphamide is an alternative for azathioprine. Not as a single agent but to use in combination with steroids (Melchionda and Harman 2019).

- If left untreated, PV can be fatal due to secondary infections and fluid and electrolyte imbalances (Baican et al. 2015).

- The mortality of PV in untreated cases or inadequately treated cases is greater than 75% (Bystryn 1996).

Table 4.1 that shows a summary of the blistering conditions discussed above and their clinical aspects that aid in their diagnosis.

Table 4.1 A summary of blistering conditions discussed and tips for their diagnosis

Blistering condition	Tips for diagnosis
Bullous pemphigoid	Tense blisters, nikolsky sign negative, oral symptoms usually are absent
Pemphigus vulgaris	Flaccid blisters, nikolsky sign positive, painful oral lesions often common Oral lesions usually precede skin lesions
Herpes simplex	Usually presents as groups of blisters around the corners of the mouth or on the genitalia Pain or tingling sensation is usually present at the site of involvement Also anywhere else on the body, if grouped vesicles are present locally, keep in mind the possibility of inoculated herpes
Herpes zoster	Pain often precedes the blisters Blistering lesions occur along the dermatome. Therefore, manifests in a ribbon shape or segmentally Lesions never cross midline
Hand foot mouth disease	Associated with a brief non-specific prodrome In addition to palms and soles, blisters can be present on sides of the feet and hands, genitalia and buttocks. Erosions noted in the oral cavity
Bullous impetigo	More common in children Tends to be more often localized Flaccid bullae
Insect bites	Can be localized or generalized History of exposure to insects may or may not always be elicited Pain could be present at the site of lesions
Contact dermatitis	Can be localized or generalized Patient can sometimes give you prior history of having similar presentation upon exposure to an offending agent such as poison ivy Presence of blisters in a linear fashion often is present

Bibliography

Baican A, Chiorean R, Leucuta DC, Baican C, Danescu S, Ciuce D, et al. Prediction of survival for patients with pemphigus vulgaris and pemphigus foliaceus: a retrospective cohort study. Orphanet J Rare Dis. 2015;10(1). Available from https://www.ncbi.nlm.nih.gov/pmc/articles/PMC4411722/pdf/13023_2015_Article_263.pdf.

Béné J, Moulis G, Bennani I, Auffret M, Coupe P, Babai S, et al. Bullous pemphigoid and dipeptidyl peptidase IV inhibitors: a case-noncase study in the French pharmacovigilance database. Br J Dermatol. 2016;175(2):296–301.

Boulard C, Duvert Lehembre S, Picard-Dahan C, Kern JS, Zambruno G, Feliciani C, et al. Calculation of cut-off values based on the autoimmune bullous skin disorder intensity score (ABSIS) and pemphigus disease area index (PDAI) pemphigus scoring systems for defining moderate, significant and extensive types of pemphigus. Br J Dermatol. 2016;175(1):142–9.

Bullous pemphigoid. Primary Care Dermatology Society. Available from https://www.pcds.org.uk/clinical-guidance/bullous-pemphigoid1.

Bystryn JC. The adjuvant therapy of pemphigus. An update. Arch Dermatol. 1996;132(2):203–12.

Cholera M, Chainani-Wu N. Management of pemphigus vulgaris. Adv Ther. 2016;33(6):910–58.

Gregoriou S, Efthymiou O, Stefanaki C, Rigopoulos D. Management of pemphigus vulgaris: challenges and solutions. Clin Cosmetic Investigational Dermatol. 2015;8:521–7. Available from https://www.ncbi.nlm.nih.gov/pmc/articles/PMC4622091/.

CDC. Hand foot and mouth disease. Centers for Disease Control and Prevention; 2019. Available from https://www.cdc.gov/hand-foot-mouth/about/signs-symptoms.html.

Joly P, Maho-Vaillant M, Prost-Squarcioni C, Hebert V, Houivet E, Calbo S, et al. First-line rituximab combined with short-term prednisone versus prednisone alone for the treatment of pemphigus (Ritux 3): a prospective, multicentre, parallel-group, open-label randomised trial. Lancet. 2017;389(10083):2031–40.

Joly P, Baricault S, Sparsa A, Bernard P, Bédane C, Duvert-Lehembre S, et al. Incidence and mortality of bullous pemphigoid in France. J Investigative Dermatol. 2012;132(8):1998–2004. Available from https://www.sciencedirect.com/science/article/pii/S0022202X15358620.

Kimmis BD, Downing C, Tyring S. Hand-foot-and-mouth disease caused by coxsackievirus A6 on the rise. PubMed. 2018;102(5):353–6.

Lamberts A, Meijer JM, Jonkman MF. Nonbullous pemphigoid: a systematic review. J Am Acad Dermatol. 2018;78(5):989-995.e2.

Malik AM, Tupchong S, Huang S, Are A, Hsu S, Motaparthi K. An updated review of pemphigus diseases. Medicina. 2021;57(10):1080.

Melchionda V, Harman KE. Pemphigus vulgaris and pemphigus foliaceus: an overview of the clinical presentation, investigations and management. Clin Exp Dermatol. 2019;44(7):740–6.

Pemphigoid B, Miyamoto D, Santi C, Aoki V, Maruta C. Continuing mediCAl eduCAtion. 2018. Available from https://www.scielo.br/pdf/abd/v94n2/0365-0596-abd-94-02-0133.pdf

Pemphigus vulgaris and pemphigus vegetans. Primary Care Dermatology Society. Available from https://www.pcds.org.uk/clinical-guidance/pemphigus-vulgaris.

Ruocco V, Sacerdoti G. Pemphigus and bullous pemphigoid due to drugs. Int J Dermatol. 1991;30(5):307–12.

Schmidt E, Obe K, Bröcker EB, Zillikens D. Serum levels of autoantibodies to BP180 correlate with disease activity in patients with bullous pemphigoid. Arch Dermatol. 2000;136(2).

Williams HC, Wojnarowska F, Kirtschig G, Mason J, Godec TR, Schmidt E, et al. Doxycycline versus prednisolone as an initial treatment strategy for bullous pemphigoid: a pragmatic, non-inferiority, randomised controlled trial. The Lancet. 2017;389(10079):1630–8.

Chapter 5
Eczema

Abstract Eczema is a common dermatological condition encountered in primary care. Broadly, eczema can be divided into exogenous and endogenous eczema based on the offending agent. In endogenous eczema, the offending agent is within the body and in exogenous eczema the offending agent is outside the body. Contact dermatitis is the prototype of the exogenous eczema. There are several types that can fall in the category of endogenous eczema. In this chapter, we will discuss the common ones among them and also about contact dermatitis. The chapter discusses mainly from their clinical perspective. It provides details about the clinical presentation of these conditions and ways to diagnose them; where feasible it provides clinical information regarding how to diagnose them clinically. It also discusses their treatment options and where appropriate the circumstances as to when the patients need to be referred to the dermatologist.

Keywords Atopic dermatitis · Seborrheic dermatitis · Pompholyx · Dyshydrotic eczema · Stasis dermatitis · Asteotic eczema · Lichen simplex chronicus · Nummular eczema · Contact dermatitis

The common types of endogenous eczema are:

- Atopic Dermatitis
- Seborrheic Dermatitis
- Pompholyx
- Stasis Dermatitis
- Asteotic Eczema
- Lichen Simplex Chronicus

D. K. Yellumahanthi, *Manual of Primary Care Dermatology*,
https://doi.org/10.1007/978-3-031-68406-7_5

– Nummular Eczema.

5.1 Atopic Dermatitis (AD)

– AD is a chronic pruritic relapsing inflammatory skin disorder.

– AD is more common in children. It could be associated with allergic rhinitis, asthma, rhino conjunctivitis and food allergies (Batllés-Garrido et al. 2010; Eller et al. 2009; Eichenfield et al. 2014).

– The clinical appearance of AD depends on age of the patient (Napolitano et al. 2022).

– Mainly facial and extensor involvement in infancy and up to two years. The clinical presentation is mainly itchy papules and vesicles with poorly defined erythema (Napolitano et al. 2022). Please see Chap. 9 “Face” Fig. 9.8, for AD on the face.

– Manifests as flexural eczema (Front of elbows and back of knees) in children and adults. The clinical picture in children is more of lichenified papules and plaques with dry skin. In adults, it is predominantly papules and plaques (Napolitano et al. 2022). Please see Chap. 11, “Upper Extremity Including Hands” Fig. 11.4 for AD involving the cubital fossa and Chap. 14, ‘Legs’ Fig. 14.7 for AD involving the popliteal fossa.

– AD may subside as the patient grows older.

– AD can occur in adults for first time as well (Silverberg et al. 2018).

– The adult onset AD can manifest as localized dermatitis, such as hand dermatitis, nipple, or eyelid eczema. Also the picture of AD in adults could vary a lot (Langan et al. 2020; Girolomoni et al. 2021).

5.1.1 Diagnosis

– Although there are various guidelines consisting of major and minor criteria for diagnosis of AD, given its varied presentation, often the physician’s assessment made clinically is considered as the gold standard for diagnosis of AD (Krol and Krafchik 2006). The classical distribution of lesions in the sites discussed above, the history of recurrences and the presence of associated clinical conditions should alert a clinician regarding the suspicion of diagnosis of AD.

5.1.2 Management

- Given the chronicity of AD, having a child with moderate to severe AD could have a profound impact on the social and emotional perspectives of families (Langan et al. 2020; Strathie Page et al. 2016).

  Therefore, effective treatment not only improves the quality of the child's life but also helps the entire family as a whole.

- Education, excellent skin care, avoidance of irritants and allergens, and treating inflammation are the key components of the management.

Education:

- Education has a pivotal role to play in its management. Patient education is important for the prognosis of AD in children. Most guidelines reiterated that patient education has proven results in reducing the severity of the disease, improving both mental health and overall quality of life as well (Wollenberg et al. 2018).

- It is important for parents to get educated on the nature of the disease and the goals of therapy. Understanding the chronic, relapsing nature of AD is important, as is counseling on the prognosis and natural history.

Emolients:

- The gist of basic skin care is to make sure skin is well hydrated.

- Skin moisturization, along with cleaning can reduce the severity of AD and also can benefit by reducing the frequency of medication use (Katibi et al. 2022).

- Numerous emollients are available that are suitable for use on atopic dry skin. In general, ointments and creams are more effective than lotions.

Avoidance of irritants and allergens:

- Any known triggers for a given patient needs to be avoided. Lukewarm quick baths, usage of unscented soaps and wearing 100% cotton clothing can all help in avoiding irritants. Also, making sure one's skin is well hydrated also helps as dry skin has a low threshold to get irritated easily.

Anti-inflammatory agents:

- Topical steroids are usually the first drugs of choice prescribed by physicians to reduce the inflammation/eczema.

- If possible in children avoid usage of topical steroids in sensitive areas, such as the face and neck, to avoid the potential side effects associated with their usage (Wang et al. 2022).

- Mild potency steroids such as desonide 0.05% cream are to be used for the face if needed (except eyelid). For eyelids, topical calcineurin agents such tacroliums and pimecrolimus can be used.

- More potent topical steroids can be used for the other body sites to treat the flare-ups. For instance, on the body other than face, depending on the severity, moderate potent agents such as hydrocortisone valerate 0.2% ointment or potent agents such as betamethasone dipropionate 0.05% ointment can be used. From author's point of view, in general, it is prudent to avoid using topical steroids for more than two weeks at a stretch. If needed, they can be resumed after a gap of about two weeks.

- Step down treatment can be done using topical calcineurin inhibitors like pimecrolimus and tacrolimus.

- Pimecrolimus 1% cream can be used for mild-to moderate AD. Tacrolimus ointment (0.03% or 0.1%) can be used for treating moderate-to-severe AD. Both pimecrolimus and tacrolimus are approved for ages 2 years and older in the United States (Butala and Paller 2022).

- Topical crisaborole is also an alternative. It can be used in the treatment of mild to moderate AD in patients 3 months and older (Paller et al. 2016; Schlessinger et al. 2020; Eichenfield et al. 2017).

- Topical roflumilast, a phosphodiesterase 4 inhibitor, 0.15% cream has been approved recently for mild-moderate AD for 6years and older patients (Roflumilast cream).

- Ruxolitinib 1.5% cream, a janus kinase (JAK) inhibitor has been approval for patients 12 years old and older with mild-to-moderate AD (Butala and Paller 2022).

- **Systemic treatment**: The decision to start systematic treatment could depend not only on the severity of the disease but also factors such as risks and benefits of treatment and its impact on quality of life, and risks and benefits of systematic treatments for each patient (Simpson et al. 2017).

  There are several options for systemic treatment, and they include oral steroids, cyclosporin A, azathioprine, methotrexate and dupilumab, an interleukin-4 receptor inhibitor.

  Systemic steroids for prolonged use are discouraged. Oral prednisone treatment is usually not recommended for more than 2 weeks (Boguniewicz et al. 2017).

There is limited evidence of effectiveness of antihistamines in treating pruritus, so most guidelines do not recommend their systemic usage (Wang et al. 2022).

- In general, if AD is not controlled with standard topical measures, recommend referring to a dermatologist for further management.

5.2 Seborrheic Dermatitis

- About 1–3% of the adult population is affected with seborrheic dermatitis (Borda and Wikramanayake 2015).

- The exact etiology is multifactorial. Malasseizia, the normal body yeast is the likely the cause of seborrheic dermatitis (Gemmer et al. 2002).

- Dandruff is a mildest form of seborrheic dermatitis. It differs from other degrees of seborrheic dermatitis by being devoid of any erythema. It is manifested on the scalp purely as fine, white, diffuse scaliness without any underlying erythema (Bouillon 2005).

- Apart from its mildest form, seborrheic dermatitis manifests as erythematous plaques with greasy-looking scales that involves the seborrheic areas of the body such as scalp, glabella, eyebrows, nasolabial folds, post auricular region, tip of the chin, front of the chest, inter scapular area, pubic area (Figs. 5.1, 5.2 and 5.3). Please see Fig. 3.11 in Chap. 3, "Papulosqumaous Disorders" for seborrheic dermatitis involving the beard area.

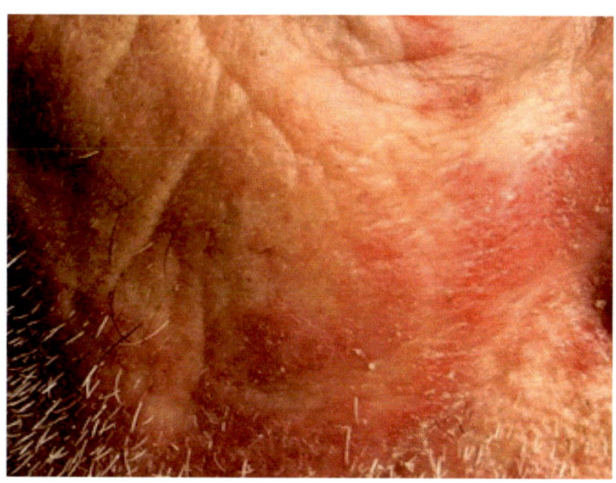

Fig. 5.1 Seborrheic dermatitis involving nasolabial folds

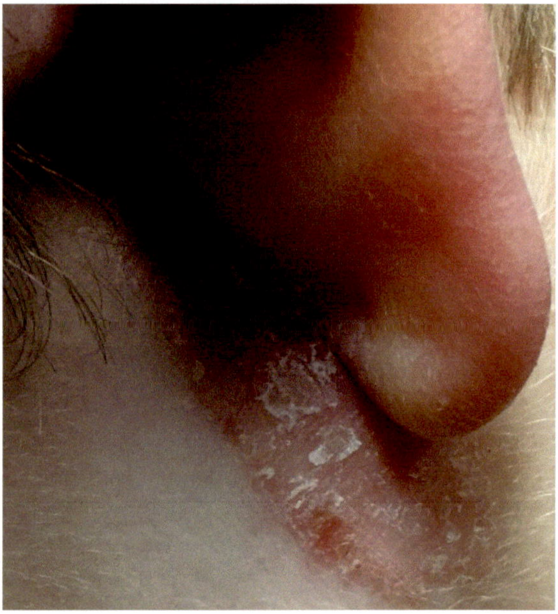

Fig. 5.2 Seborrheic dermatitis in post auricular region

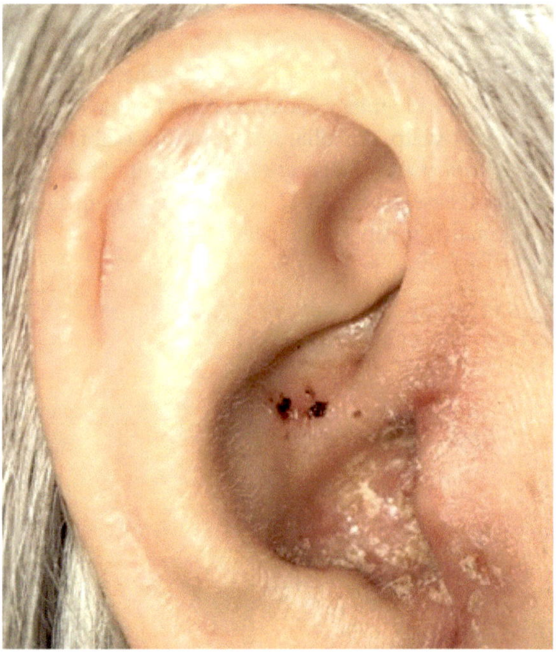

Fig. 5.3 Seborrheic dermatitis involving external ear

Fig. 5.4 Cradle cap

– Not always all the above seborrheic areas are involved. However, examination of all the above sites need to be done anytime Seborrheic dermatitis is suspected as it can help in both diagnosis and the extent of involvement. The latter can help in tailoring the treatment appropriately.

– Infants: In infants, seborrheic dermatitis commonly involves the scalp, post auricular region, axilla and diaper area. If seborrheic dermatitis is confined only to the scalp, it is called Cradle cap (Fig. 5.4).

5.2.1 Management

– It needs to be discussed with patients that there is no cure for seborrheic dermatitis and that the course is chronic with waxing and waning. The therapeutics currently used for seborrheic dermatitis help only in alleviating the symptoms.

The following are the common agents used for managing seborrheic dermatitis:

a. Zinc pyrithrone

– Can be used as first line choice of mild seborrheic dermatitis.

– Also can be used for both maintenance and prevention (Mangion et al. 2023).

b. Topical imidazoles such as ketoconazole, clotrimazole, miconazole

– Ketoconazole has better efficacy than other imidazoles (Punyani et al. 2021). Can be used for both adult and infantile seborrheic dermatitis

c. Topical steroids

– Indicated for short-term management when there is significant inflammation associated with moderate to severe seborrheic dermatitis (Mangion et al. 2023). The potency of steroids needs to be tailored as below based on the site and severity of seborrheic dermatitis.

- Seborrheic dermatitis on face: Low potency agents such as desonide 0.05% cream.

- Intertrigionous areas: Same as above.

- For seborrheic dermatitis on trunk and scalp, medium to strong potent agents such as hydrocortisone valerate 0.2% ointment or betamethasone dipropionate 0.05% ointment.

d. Topical Calcineurin inhibitors: (Tacrolimus, Pimecromilus)

- Can be used for seborrheic dermatitis when topical antifungals cannot be used, more so on the face.

e. Phosphodiesterase inhibitor

- Roflumilast, 0.3% foam has been approved recently for patients 9 years and older (Roflumilast topical foam).

- **Dandruff:** Commonly used agents are zinc pyrithrone, selenium sulfide 2.5% lotion (for mild to moderate) and ketoconazole 2% lotion.

- **For cradle cap,** usually application of emollients such as mineral oil or vaseline and usage of baby shampoos and removing scales by brushing gently with a comb should help (Waldman and Grant-Kels 2022).

- Systemic treatment for seborrheic dermatitis is generally reserved for cases that are severe or refractory. Oral terbinafine and oral fluconazole are the main systemic agents used for treating seborrheic dermatitis (Borda et al. 2019).

- Terbinafine is usually administered as daily at a dosage of 250 mg, generally over the course of 4–6 weeks (Vena et al. 2005).

- Oral fluconazole in the dose of 150 mg/weekly over 4 weeks is among the several regimens used (Zisova 2009).

5.3 Pompholyx (Dyshidrotic Eczema)

- It is characterized by recurrent itchy vesicular eruption that affects the palms, soles or both (Venkatesh et al. 2023).

5.3.1 *Diagnosis*

- Based on clinical examination Please make sure the diagnosis of pompholyx should be made only if blisters are confined to either palms or soles or both. If blisters are present elsewhere along with palms and soles, then search should be made for other diagnosis.

5.3.2 *Management*

- Topical ultra (Super) potent steroids. Topical calcineurin inhibitors and phototherapy have also been used (Venkatesh et al. 2023).

- Referral to dermatology can be done for cases refractory to topical therapy.

- Please see Chap. 11, "Upper extremity including Hands" Fig. 9 for picture of pompholyx and also to read more about its clinical features and management.

5.4 Stasis Dermatitis or Stasis Eczema

- Stasis dermatitis is a cutaneous manifestation of chronic venous insufficiency (Yosipovitch et al. 2023).

- It manifests as erythematous, eczematous plaques on the lower part of the legs (Rzepecki and Blasiak 2018).

- Usually presents bilaterally.

- Besides the dermatitis, it is characterized by symptoms such as itching, pain and swelling.

5.4.1 *Diagnosis*

- Diagnosis is usually obvious from clinical examination.

5.4.2 *Management*

- Compression therapy and leg elevation are the mainstay of treatment for the venous insufficiency; topical corticosteroids for the dermatitis. The potency of the steroid is proportional to the inflammation. Low potency steroids for mild inflammation and potent ones for severe inflammation.

– Refractory cases can be referred to vascular surgeon to see if there is any definitive therapy for the vascular insufficiency.

– Please see Chap. 14, 'Legs' Fig. 14.2 for picture of stasis dermatitis and for more details on clinical manifestations and management.

5.5 Asteatotic Eczema (Eczema Craquele)

– Asteotitc eczema is the most common type of eczema in the elderly (Polat and İlhan 2015).

– Manifests as dry, inflamed, cracked, and scaly skin (https://www.ncbi.nlm.nih.gov/books/NBK549807/).

– More common in lower extremities.

– Dryness is often the cause of this condition.

5.5.1 Management

– Application of emolients. Topical steroids for short period of times can be given if needed.

– Also, please see Chap. 14, 'Legs' Fig. 14.6 for picture of asteatotic eczema and more details on clinical features and management.

5.6 Nummular Eczema (Nummular Dermatitis) (Discoid Eczema)

– Manifests as coin shaped eczematous patches or plaques on extremities.

– Symmetrical presentation is common

5.6.1 Diagnosis

– The coin shape of the eczematous lesions and the presence on extremities should help in the diagnosis.

5.6.2 Management

– Potent steroids such as betamethasone dipropionate 0.05%ointment.

– Please see Chap. 14, 'Legs' Fig. 14.5 and Chap. 11 'Upper Extremity Including Hands' Fig. 11.5 for pictures of nummular eczema and more details on its clinical features and management.

5.7 Exogenous Eczema

– Contact dermatitis is the prototype of exogenous eczema.

5.7.1 Contact Dermatitis

– Contact Dermatitis needs to be considered in the differential diagnosis of all the skin rashes.

– On the scalp, hair dyes; on the face all cosmetics; in the axilla deodorant are the common ones that need to be suspected. Please see Chap. 12, 'Axilla' Figs. 12.1 and 12.2 for picture of contact dermatitis likely to deodorant.

– Airborne allergens can also cause contact dermatitis on the face.

– The pattern of skin rash secondary to contact dermatitis is based on the cause of exposure and the involved body part. For instance, cosmetics could be the culprit if both cheeks are involved, hair dyes could be the offending allergen if upper part of the forehead close to the hairline is involved. Upper eyelids, nasolabial folds, and chin area can involve with airborne allergens (Waldman and Grant-Kels 2022).

– Nickel allergy is very common. Among many others, nickel is an ingredient in the jean buttons, bra hooks and some jewelry. Therefore, any rashes that are in the vicinity of bra hooks, jean buttons, ear lobes, sides of the neck need to be ruled out for nickel allergy.

- Please see Chap. 10, ‘Trunk’ Fig. 10.9 for picture of contact dermatitis to jean button. Likely due to nickel allergy.

- Contact dermatitis to clothing typically occurs in body areas where there is most friction—axilla, inner aspects of upper extremities, medial side of thighs.

- Contact dermatitis to poison ivy occurs in the areas of contact and is quite commonly encountered. Lesions in a linear morphology is often a clue that there was a contact with an exogenous allergen such as poison ivy (Fig. 5.5).

- Contact dermatitis to topical medications can also occur (Fig. 5.6).

- Generalized rashes can also be caused by contact dermatitis. Any bizarre looking rash, please make sure contact dermatitis is ruled out.

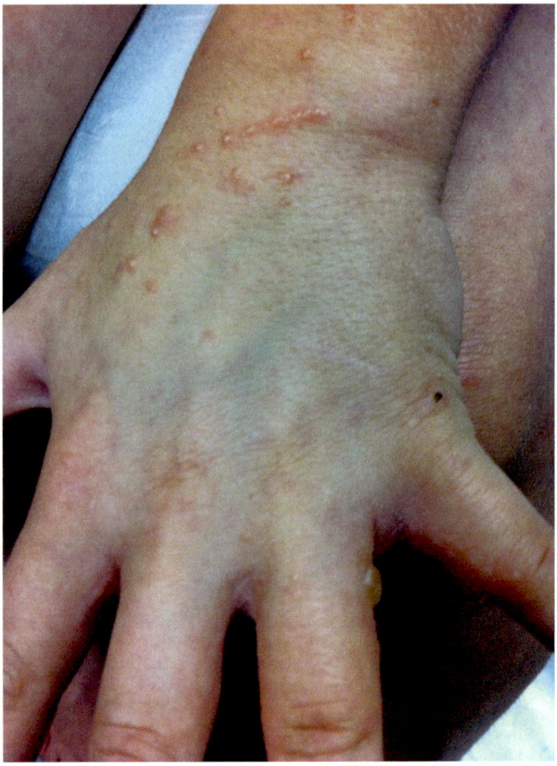

Fig. 5.5 Contact dermatitis to poison ivy. Please note near the wrist lesions in a linear morphology

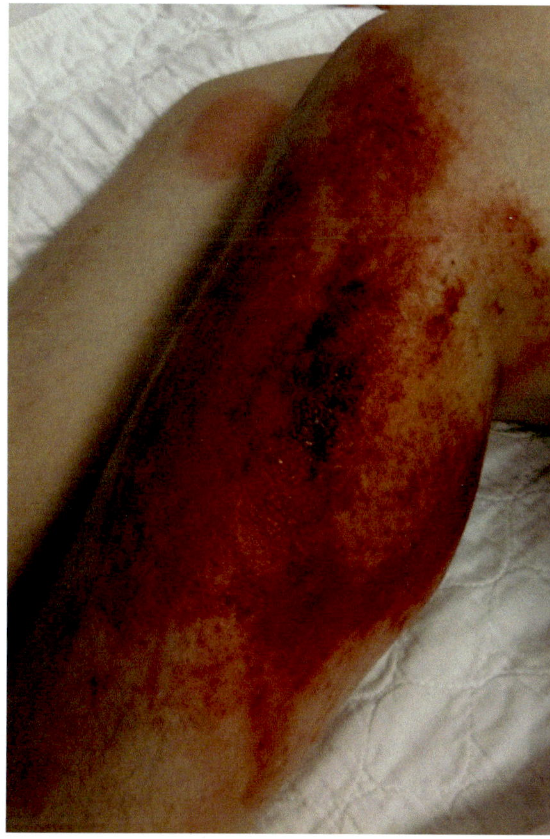

Fig. 5.6 Contact dermatitis to topical medicament

Management

- Identifying and avoiding the potential allergen is the first and foremost important step in the management of contact dermatitis.

- Often it is difficult to identify the offending allergen and a detailed history needs to be obtained.

- Also it needs to be kept in mind, not always patients tend to develop contact dermatitis to a new object/substance they came in contact. Sometimes, patient may be using something for a long time and may have tolerated it until recently when they may have started developing contact dermatitis to it.

- Topical glucocorticoids are often the drugs used towards management. Depending on the body area, appropriate topical steroids can be given: For instance, on the face, desonide 0.05% cream, on the body other than face, depending on the severity, either medium potent steroid such as hydrocortisone valerate 0.2% ointment or potent steroid such as betamethasone dipropionate 0.05% ointment. Systemic steroids for a short duration can be given if the inflammation is extensive.

– Cases where, contact dermatitis is suspected but potential allergen cannot be identified, need to be referred to a dermatologist for a possible patch testing and for further management.

Bibliography

Borda LJ, Wikramanayake TC. Seborrheic dermatitis and dandruff: a comprehensive review. J Clin Investigative Dermatol. 2015;3(2).

Borda LJ, Perper M, Keri JE. Treatment of seborrheic dermatitis: a comprehensive review. J Dermatol Treatment. 2019;30(2):158–69. Available from https://www.ncbi.nlm.nih.gov/pubmed/29737895

Bouillon C. The science of hair care. 2nd ed. 2005.

Butala S, Paller AS. Optimizing topical management of atopic dermatitis. Ann Allergy Asthma Immunol. 2022;128(5):488–504.

Eichenfield LF, Call RS, Forsha DW, Fowler J, Hebert AA, Spellman M, et al. Long-term safety of crisaborole ointment 2% in children and adults with mild to moderate atopic dermatitis. J Am Acad Dermatol. 2017;77(4):641–649.e5. Available from https://pubmed.ncbi.nlm.nih.gov/28823881/.

Eller E, Kjaer HF, Høst A, Andersen KE, Bindslev-Jensen C. Food allergy and food sensitization in early childhood: results from the DARC cohort. Allergy. 2009;64(7):1023–9.

Batllés-Garrido J, Torres-Borrego J, Rubí-Ruiz T, Bonillo-Perales A, González-Jiménez Y, Momblán-De Cabo J, et al. Prevalence and factors linked to allergic rhinitis in 10 and 11-year-old children in Almería. Isaac Phase II, Spain. PubMed. 2010;38(3):135–41.

Paller AS, Tom WL, Lebwohl MG, Blumenthal RL, Boguniewicz M, Call RS, et al. Efficacy and safety of crisaborole ointment, a novel, nonsteroidal phosphodiesterase 4 (PDE4) inhibitor for the topical treatment of atopic dermatitis (AD) in children and adults. J Am Acad Dermatol. 2016;75(3):494–503.e6. Available from https://www.jaad.org/action/showPdf?pii=S0190-9622%2816%2930330-9.

Boguniewicz M, Alexis AF, Beck LA, Block J, Eichenfield LF, Fonacier L, et al. Expert perspectives on management of moderate-to-severe atopic dermatitis: a multidisciplinary consensus addressing current and emerging therapies. J Allergy Clin Immunolo Practice. 2017;5(6):1519–31. Available from https://www.scholars.northwestern.edu/en/publications/expert-perspectives-on-management-of-moderate-to-severe-atopic-de.

Silverberg JI, Vakharia PP, Chopra R, Sacotte R, Patel N, Immaneni S, et al. Phenotypical differences of childhood- and adult-onset atopic dermatitis. J Allergy Clin Immunol Practice. 2018;6(4):1306–12.

Langan SM, Irvine AD, Weidinger S. Atopic dermatitis. Lancet. 2020;396(10247):345–60.7.

Napolitano M, Fabbrocini G, Martora F, Genco L, Noto M, Patruno C. Children atopic dermatitis: diagnosis, mimics, overlaps, and therapeutic implication. Dermatol Therapy. 2022;35(12).

Venkatesh S, Fakhraie S, Chovatiya R. Recalcitrant dyshidrotic eczema successfully treated with upadacitinib. Dermatitis®. 2023.

.Yosipovitch G, Mark Jackson J, Nedorost ST, Friedman A, Adiri R, Cha A, et al. Stasis dermatitis: the burden of disease, diagnosis, and treatment. Dermatitis. 2023.

https://www.ncbi.nlm.nih.gov/books/NBK549807/

Eichenfield LF, Tom WL, Berger TG, Krol A, Paller AS, Schwarzenberger K, et al. Guidelines of care for the management of atopic dermatitis: section 2. Management and treatment of atopic dermatitis with topical therapies. J Am Acad Dermatol. 2014;71(1):116–32. Available from https://www.ncbi.nlm.nih.gov/pubmed/24813302.

Gemmer CM, DeAngelis YM, Theelen B, Boekhout T, Dawson TL. Fast, noninvasive method for molecular detection and differentiation of malassezia yeast species on human skin and application of the method to dandruff microbiology. J Clin Microbiol. 2002;40(9):3350–7.

Girolomoni G, de Bruin-Weller M, Aoki V, Kabashima K, Deleuran M, Puig L, et al. Nomenclature and clinical phenotypes of atopic dermatitis. Therapeutic Adv Chronic Dis. 2021;12:204062232110029.

Katibi OS, Cork MJ, Flohr C, Danby SG. Moisturizer therapy in prevention of atopic dermatitis and food allergy: to use or disuse? Ann Allergy Asthma Immunol. 2022;128(5):512–25.

Krol A, Krafchik B. The differential diagnosis of atopic dermatitis in childhood. Dermatol Ther. 2006;19(2):73–82. Available from https://www.ncbi.nlm.nih.gov/pubmed/16669989.

Mangion SE, Mackenzie L, Roberts MS, Holmes AM. Seborrheic dermatitis: topical therapeutics and formulation design. Euro J Pharmaceut Biopharmaceut. 2023;185:148–64. Available from https://www.sciencedirect.com/science/article/pii/S0939641123000292?casa_token=mTq2uXFjItoAAAAA:s9mKF9tFlYPx46ec4ftQeXDx3f-cZVSv70E4--m7vzm2zO6HtxO0La5fj5eSECd2i3Tuj0VCoYY.

Polat M, İlhan MN. Dermatological complaints of the elderly attending a dermatology outpatient clinic in Turkey: a prospective study over a one-year period. PubMed. 2015;23(4):277–81.

Punyani S, Tosti A, Hordinsky M, Yeomans D, Schwartz J. The impact of shampoo wash frequency on scalp and hair conditions. Skin Appendage Disorders. 2021;7(3):1–11.

Roflumilast cream, 0.15%. US Food and Drug Administration. Supplemental new drug application. https://www.accessdata.fda.gov/drugsatfda_docs/appletter/2024/215985Orig1s007ltr.pdf

Roflumilast topical foam, 0.3%. US Food and Drug Administration (FDA) approved product information. Revised December 2023. US Food and Drug Administration. https://www.accessdata.fda.gov/drugsatfda_docs/label/2023/217242s000lbl.pdf

Rzepecki AK, Blasiak R. Stasis dermatitis: differentiation from other common causes of lower leg inflammation and management strategies. Curr Geriatrics Rep. 2018;7(4):222–7.

Schlessinger J, Shepard JS, Gower R, Su JC, Lynde C, Cha A, et al. Safety, effectiveness, and pharmacokinetics of crisaborole in infants aged 3 to < 24 months with mild-to-moderate atopic dermatitis: a phase IV open-label study (CrisADe CARE 1). Am J Clin Dermatol. 2020;21(2):275–84. Available from https://www.ncbi.nlm.nih.gov/pmc/articles/PMC7125059.

Simpson EL, Bruin-Weller M, Flohr C, Ardern-Jones MR, Barbarot S, Deleuran M, et al. When does atopic dermatitis warrant systemic therapy? Recommendations from an expert panel of the International Eczema Council. J Am Acad Dermatol. 2017;77(4):623–33.

Strathie Page S, Weston S, Loh R. Atopic dermatitis in children. Aust Fam Physician. 2016;45(5):293–6.

Vena GA, Micali G, Santoianni P, Cassano N, Peruzzi E. Oral terbinafine in the treatment of multi-site seborrheic dermatitis: a multicenter, double-blind placebo-controlled study. Int J Immunopathol Pharmacol. 2005;18(4):745–53.

Waldman RA, Grant-Kels JM. Dermatology for the primary care provider. Philadelphia, PA: Elsevier; 2022.

Wang Q, Liu L, Gao S, Su S. Guidelines for the management of atopic dermatitis in children: a systematic review. Int Arch Allergy Immunol. 2022;184(2):132–41.

Wollenberg A, Barbarot S, Bieber T, Christen-Zaech S, Deleuran M, Fink-Wagner A, et al. Consensus-based European guidelines for treatment of atopic eczema (atopic dermatitis) in adults and children: part I. J Eur Acad Dermatol Venereol. 2018;32(5):657–82.

Zisova LG. Treatment of Malassezia species associated seborrheic blepharitis with fluconazole. PubMed. 2009;51(3):57–9.

Chapter 6
Common Cutaneous Infections

Abstract This chapter provides an overview of the common cutaneous infections caused mainly by bacteria, fungi and viruses. The chapter discusses mainly from their clinical perspective. It provides details about the clinical presentation of these conditions and ways to diagnose them; when feasible, it provides clinical information regarding how to diagnose them clinically. It also discusses their treatment options and the circumstances as to when the patients need to be referred to the dermatologist.

Keywords Folliculitis · Impetigo · Molluscum Contagiosum · Warts · Verruca vulgaris · Tinea · Candidiasis · Herpes simplex labialis · Herpes genitalis · Herpes zoster · Furuncle · Carbuncle · Abscess · Cellulitis · Scabies

In this chapter, we will discuss clinical manifestations, diagnosis and management of common infections.

Bacterial: impetigo.

Folliculitis.
Furuncle.
Carbuncle.
Abscess.
Cellulitis.
Erythrasma.

Viral: Molluscum contagiosum.

Herpes simplex labialis.
Herpes genitalis.
Herpes zoster.
Verruca vulgaris.

Fungal: dermatophytosis.
Cutaneous candidiasis.

Miscellaneous: scabies.

D. K. Yellumahanthi, *Manual of Primary Care Dermatology*,
https://doi.org/10.1007/978-3-031-68406-7_6

Bacterial Infections

Impetigo.
Folliculitis.
Furuncle.
Carbuncle.
Abscess.
Cellulitis.
Erythrasma.

6.1 Impetigo

- It commonly occurs in children. Two clinical types are present. Non-bullous (or impetigo contagiosa) and bullous impetigo.

- **Non-bullous impetigo** (Fig. 6.1) is the more common one accounting for 70% of all impetigo (Preda-Naumescu et al. 2021).

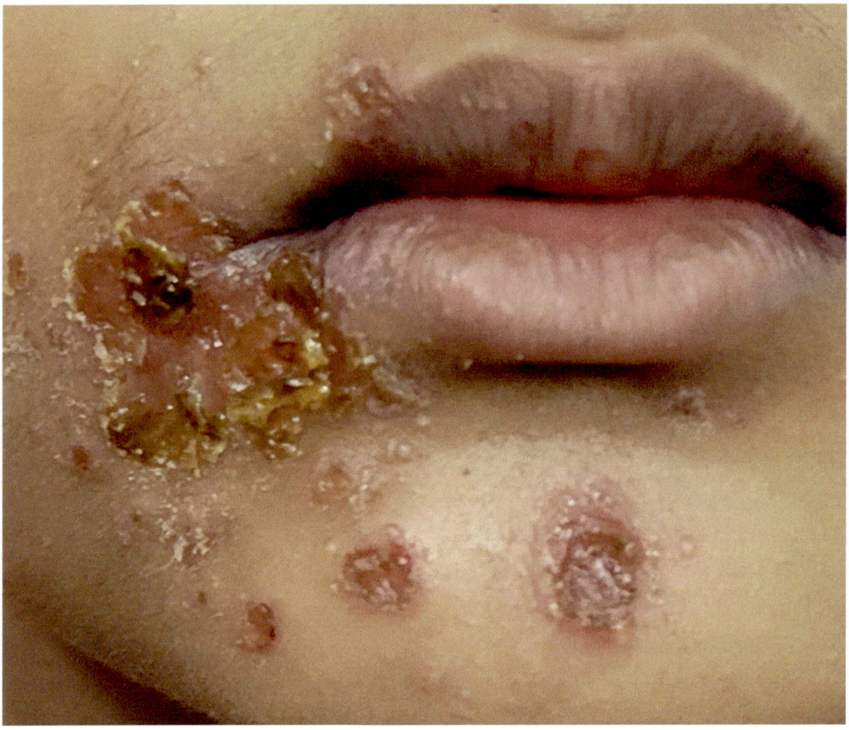

Fig. 6.1 Impetigo. *Courtesy* Dr. P.V. Krishna Rao, Dermatologist, India

- It is often caused by *Staphylococci aureus* (*S. aureus*). Group A streptococci can also cause.
- Extremities and face are commonly involved (Chiller et al. 2020).
- The initial lesions are erythematous papules that become vesicles and pustules, which upon rupture leave honey-colored crusted papules on an erythematous base.
- **Bullous impetigo** is caused by *Staphylococci aureus*. Most common age group: 2–5 years (Preda-Naumescu et al. 2021).
- Common areas: Diaper area, neck and axilla (Ibrahim et al. 2015).
- Flaccid bullae arise on apparently normal skin. Upon rupturing leaves a crusted and erythematous lesion.
- While lymphadenopathy can occur with non-bullous type, lymphadenopathy with bullous impetigo is rare (Ibrahim et al. 2015).

6.1.1 Diagnosis

- Evident clinically. Honey-colored crusts are a clue for impetigo contagiosa. When in doubt, gram stain and culture of the exudate can help in identifying the organism.

6.1.2 Management

- Impetigo (non-bullous and bullous) can be treated with topical antibiotics if lesions are localized. Topical antibiotics include mupirocin 2% topical ointment or retapamulin 1% ointment. Neomycin, bacitracin and fusidic acid can also be used (Stevens et al. 2014).
- Gentle physical removal of the superficial crusts by cleansing with soap and water or saline soaks can be used as adjunctive supportive measures.
- If extensive areas are involved or systemic signs are present, oral antibiotics may be needed (Stevens et al. 2014).

- Drugs that are active against methicillin-sensitive Staphylococcus aureus (MSSA) are usually effective unless methicillin-resistant Staphylococcus aureus (MRSA) is suspected. Commonly prescribed one is cephalexin. Erythromycin is an alternative in those who are allergic to penicillin.

- If MRSA is suspected, trimethoprim-sulfamethoxazole and clindamycin are the common antibiotic that can be used.

6.2 Folliculitis

- Infectious folliculitis is commonly caused by bacteria such as Staphylococcus aureus, streptococcus, Pseudomonas aeruginosa and Gram-negative bacteria (Gao et al. 2022).

- Clinically manifests as inflamed follicular papules and follicular pustules.

- Deep bacterial folliculitis in the beard area is called folliculitis barbae or sycosis barbae. Staphylococcus aureus is the usual causative organism.

6.2.1 Diagnosis

- Diagnosis is usually made on clinical grounds. Gram stain and culture can help.

6.2.2 Management

- Folliculitis can also be treated with the same regimen as that of impetigo.

- Note: Pseudofolliculitis barbae is the name given to the papules that are caused due to ingrowing of the curved shaft of the hair, more so in African American males. It usually occurs in the lower beard area. Please read the Chap. 9, on 'Face', for more details on the clinical manifestations and management of pseudofolliculitis barbae.

6.3 Furuncle (Boil): (Fig. 6.2)

– It is caused by Staphylococcus aureus.

– It develops around a hair follicle as a tender deep-seated inflammatory nodule.

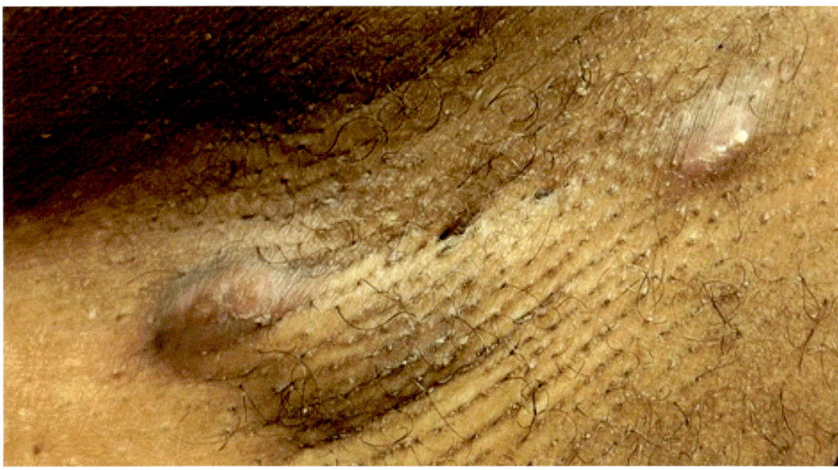

Fig. 6.2 Furuncles

6.3.1 Management

– Small furuncles can be treated with hot compresses. For larger ones, incision and drainage is needed. In addition to it, some cases may require oral antibiotics. Normally, antibiotics effective against MSSA such as cephalexin or dicloxacillin or amoxicillin and clavulanate should suffice. If methicillin-resistant Staphylococcus aureus (MRSA) is suspected, clindamycin or trimethoprim-sulfamethoxazole or doxycycline are commonly given.

6.4 Carbuncle and Abscess

6.4.1 Carbuncle

– Carbuncle manifest as deep suppurating mass. It is a deep abscesses formed in a group of adjoining follicles (Gawkrodger and Ardern-Jones 2017).

- Presents as very painful lesion that is indurated and red. There could be multiple draining pustules on its surface. Systemic symptoms such as fever and malaise may be associated

- Common areas are nape of the neck, thighs, back of the trunk (Miller 2019).

6.4.2 Abscess (Fig. 6.3)

- It is a pus-filled cavity. Either folliculitis or furuncle or carbuncle can lead to an abscess

- MRSA is usually the culprit organism.

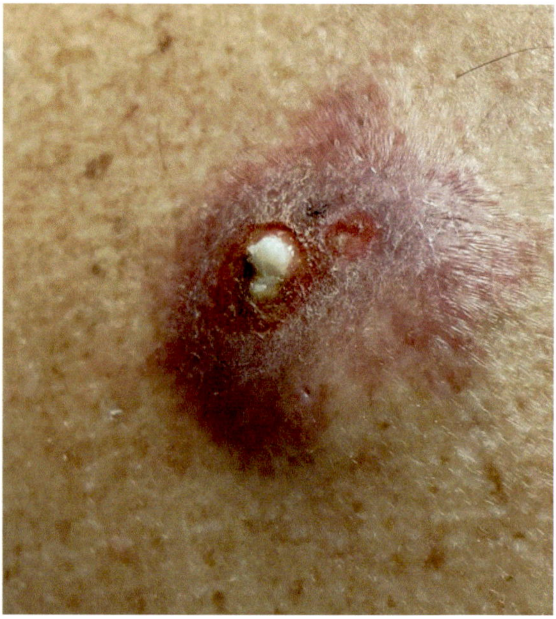

Fig. 6.3 Abscess

6.4.3 Management

- The initial management of carbuncles and abscesses is with incision and drainage.

- If MRSA is suspected, the antibiotics that can be prescribed include clindamycin and trimethoprim- sulfamethaxazole.

– For MSSA, antibiotics prescribed include dicloxacillin, cephalexin and erythromycin.

– The discharge from the lesion needs to be sent for bacterial culture and the treatment needs to be tailored as per the culture and sensitivity results.

– The topical antibiotics that can be given include mupirocin, niacin, bacitracin and fusidic acid.

– Severe or larger carbuncles and abscesses need urgent referral to a surgeon for management.

6.5 Cellulitis

– Cellulitis is the term given to the infection of the deep dermis and subcutaneous fat or tissues (Bystritsky 2021).

– Cellulitis can be purulent and non-purulent (Fig. 6.4).

– **Purulent cellulitis** (Fig. 6.5) is associated with either purulent discharge, pustule or abscess.

– **Non-purulent cellulitis** is commonly caused by Gram-positive organisms. Beta-hemolytic streptococci is the predominant one (Bystritsky 2021).

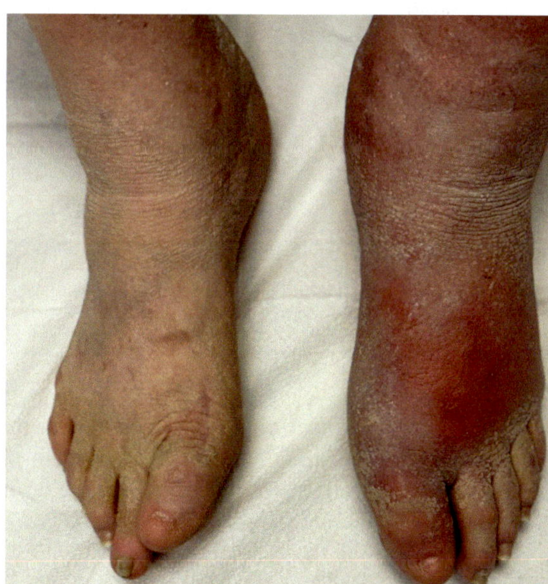

Fig. 6.4 Non-purulent cellulitis

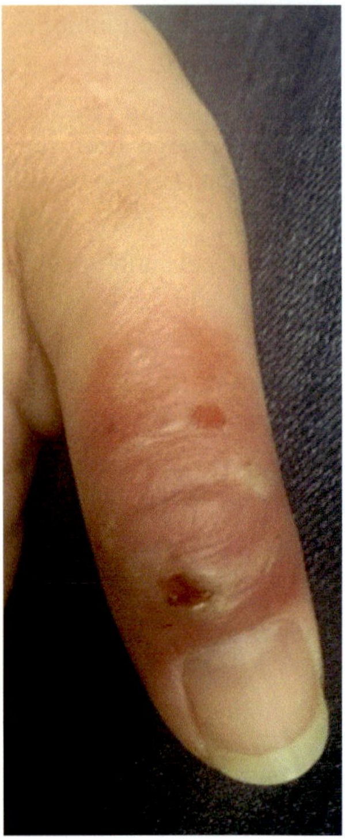

Fig. 6.5 Purulent cellulitis

- MRSA could be the common organisms causing purulent cellulitis (Moran et al. 2006).
- Cellulitis is characterized by erythema, swelling, warmth and pain of the affected site.
- Lower extremity is a common site in adults. Laterality is usually unilateral. A diagnosis of bilateral cellulitis should be made cautiously.
- Systemic symptoms are usually absent (Pearson et al.).

6.5.1 Diagnosis

- Diagnosis is often made clinically. Deep venous thrombosis (DVT) comes in the differential diagnosis. DVT tends to be more painful, and there could be some risk factors for DVT such as recent hospitalization or immobility, previous history of blood clots.When in doubt, an ultrasound of venous Doppler can be ordered to rule out DVT.

6.5.2 Management

- Includes administration of antibiotics.

- Outpatient therapy with oral antibiotics may suffice in hemodynamically stable patients with no systemic infection. On the other hand, hospitalization may be needed in the immunocompromised patients, those with severe systemic symptoms or those who failed outpatient therapy (Pearson et al.).

- In mild non-purulent cases, cephalexin or amoxicillin and clavulanate, marcolides or dicloxacillin can be given.

- In purulent cases, incision and drainage are to be done and the discharge is to be sent for culture and sensitivity. Treatment is as per the results of the culture and sensitivity. While waiting on the culture, if MRSA is suspected clindamycin or trimethoprim-sulfamethoxazole are among those drugs that can be prescribed. Newer oral agents such as delafloxacin, tedizolid and omadacycline that provide MRSA coverage should be used when other commoner ones cannot be used (Bystritsky 2021). For MSSA, cephalexin or dicloxacillin are among the antibiotics that can be given.

- Patients need to be closely monitored. If they are failing outpatient therapy or developing systemic symptoms, they need to be admitted to the hospital for further management.

- Please note if there is any underlying tinea pedis, it needs to be treated to prevent recurrent episodes of cellulitis.

6.6 Erythrasma

- The etiologic agent is *Corynebacterium minutissimum*.

- Erythrasma is manifested by well-defined but irregular reddish-brown patches, occurring in the intertriginous areas. In the toe webs, it is characterized by fissuring and white maceration.

- Common sites are the web spaces between 3rd and 4th toes, 4th and 5th toes and the inguinal folds. However, any intertriginous area can be involved (Hordinsky and Soutor 2022).

- Mostly asymptomatic or causes minimal itching.

6.6.1 *Diagnosis*

- The diagnosis is suggested by the location and clinical features described above and can be confirmed by demonstration of the characteristic coral-red fluorescence with Wood's lamp illumination.

6.6.2 *Treatment*

- Treatment includes topical clindamycin or erythromycin or azole creams. For extensive lesions, or cases not responding to topical therapy, a two-week course of oral erythromycin 250 mg po qid is effective in adults. A single dose of one gram clarithromycin is an alternative. Oral tetracycline is also effective (Blaise et al. 2008; Holdiness 2002).

- Please see Chap. 12, 'Axilla', Fig. 12.5 and Chap. 13, 'Genitals and Groin', Fig. 6.2 for pictures of erythrasma and for more details on its management.

Viral Infections

Molluscum Contagiosum.
Herpes simplex labialis.
Herpes genitalis.
Herpes zoster.
Verruca vulgaris (Warts).

6.7 Molluscum Contagiosum (MC) (Fig. 6.6)

- The causative organism for MC is a poxvirus of the Molluscipox genus (Leung 2017).

- Molluscum Contagiosum is a self-limited cutaneous viral infection.

- Usually manifests as firm, dome-shaped, umbilicated pearly papules. Could be solitary or multiple.

- More common in children and sexually active adults.

- Any site can be affected.

- Autoinoculation can occur through touching the lesion or scratching it.

- The course is self-limiting in healthy individuals. Although any given lesion lasts for about 2 months, the total duration of infection lasts longer due to spread by autoinoculation (Chen et al. 2013).

- It can last several months to more than one year also before it undergoes spontaneous regression (Gottlieb 1994). Often heals without scarring.

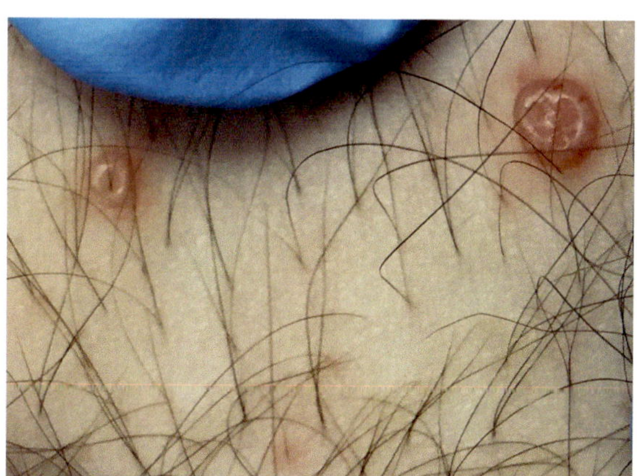

Fig. 6.6 Molluscum Contagiosum

6.7.1 Diagnosis

– Diagnosis is based on the clinical manifestations discussed.

6.7.2 Management

– Although several treatment modalities are used, no single treatment is convincingly effective (Lisette et al 2009). Therefore, 'No treatment' is also an option as it is self-limiting.

– Cryosurgery, curettage, electrodessication can be used as treatment modalities. Topical retinoids and imiquimod 5% cream can also be effective. Clinician applied topical cantharidin is also an option. It is often the treatment of choice in children as it is painless when applied (Haddock et al. 2019).

– Given that MC heals without scarring, it is important to use destructive treatments as last resort as they can cause scarring. While cryosurgery, curettage, electrodessication are the examples of destructive therapy, topical imiquimod 5% cream (immunomodulatory agent) is an example of non-destructive therapy.

6.8 Herpes Simplex

– Herpes simplex is a viral infection caused by the herpes simplex virus (HSV). There are two types of HSV: HSV-1 and HSV-2. HSV-1 is associated primarily with oral infections (Herpes labialis) (Fig. 6.7), and HSV-2 mainly genital infections. However, either type can infect any site.

– After the primary infection, HSV enters the nerve endings in the skin directly below the lesions and ascends to the dorsal root ganglia, where it remains in a dormant stage until it is reactivated.

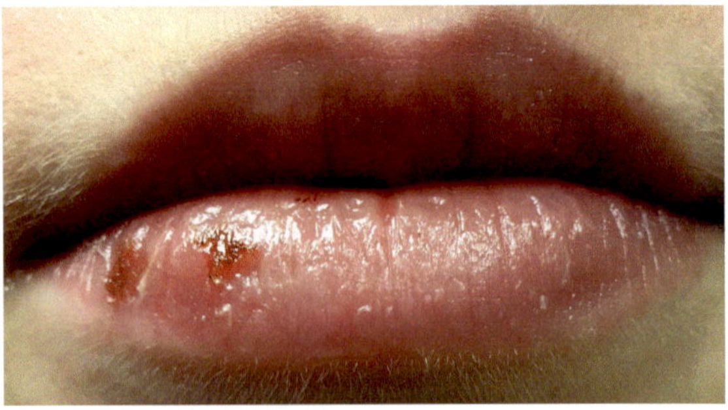

Fig. 6.7 Herpes simplex labialis

– Both herpes labialis and genitalis are chronic conditions that are associated with relapses and remissions.

6.8.1 Clinical Features

– The clinical manifestations of HSV infection vary depending on the immune status of the host and the site of infection (Cohen 2019).

Primary HSV-1 and Primary Genital Herpes

Primary HSV-1 infection:

– Primary HSV-1 infection is often associated with herpetic gingivostomatitis and pharyngitis, although it can be asymptomatic in some cases.

– Herpetic gingivostomatitis usually manifests with prodromal symptoms such as fever, myalgia, malaise, cervical or submandibular lymphadenopathy (Yarom et al. 2005).

– Initially, it is followed with hyperemia of the oral and perioral mucosa. Subsequently, eruption of vesicles follows. Vesicles ulcerate and eventually rupture. Vesicles are commonly seen on the gingiva, buccal mucosa and palate. The overall clinical picture can mimic that of aphthous stomatitis. After about 2–3 weeks, the ulcers usually heal without scarring (Aslanova et al. 2024).

Primary genital herpes:

– Vesicles, pustules and erythematous ulcers can all be seen.

– In males, the lesions commonly involve glans penis or the penile shaft or prepuce, and in females, lesions may affect the vulva, vagina or cervix (Omarova et al. 2022).

– There could be accompanying pain, dysuria and tender inguinal lymphadenopathy (Fleming et al. 2006).

– Systemic symptoms are common and include fever, headache, malaise and myalgias (Johnston et al. 2008).

Recurrent Episodes of HSV-1 (Herpes Labialis) and Recurrent Genital Herpes

– Most recurrences are not symptomatic. Symptomatic recurrences are milder than symptomatic primary infections. In general, recurrent oral infections are less symptomatic and of short duration than genital herpes.

- Recurrent genital herpes episodes usually precede with a prodrome of focal tingling or burning followed by eruption of grouped vesicles (Sauerbrei 2006).
- It typically lasts 7–10 days (Omarova et al. 2022).
- Recurrent genital herpes could occur in extragenital sites such as groin, thighs and buttocks (Cohen 2019).
- It is important to note that viral shedding can occur even during asymptomatic phase. Most of these infections are transmitted during this asymptomatic phase (Centers for Disease Control and Prevention 2022).

6.8.2 Diagnosis of Herpes Simplex

- Diagnosis is often made clinically. Where lesions are present and diagnosis is doubtful based on clinical examination, nucleic acid amplifying testing (NAAT) or culture testing can be done to confirm clinical suspicion of herpes.
- However, if these tests do not detect any virus, it does not always indicate absence of HSV infection as viral shedding is known to be intermittent (Centers for Disease Control and Prevention 2022).

6.8.3 Management

- Patients need to be educated about the chronic nature of the diagnosis.
- The role of antiviral medications is mainly to treat or prevent symptomatic outbreaks. They can also suppress the virus to reduce chances of transmission to sexual partners.
- Primary HSV gingivostomatitis is preferably treated with oral acyclovir (Cohen 2019).
- Recurrent episodes of herpes labialis, primary herpes genitalis and recurrent episodes of herpes genitalis can be treated with acyclovir or valacyclovir or famciclovir. Regimens and dosages vary with the clinical scenario (Table 6.1).
- Usually recurrent oral infections are less symptomatic and of short duration than genital herpes. Antiviral therapy hastens healing and shortens the duration of pain and discomfort of these lesions. Antiviral treatment needs to be administered ideally in the prodromal stage or within 48 h from the onset of lesions to achieve optimal results (Leung and Barankin 2017).

Table 6.1 Some of the oral regimens for herpes in immunocompetent adults

Initial HSV-1 (Cohen 2019)	**Initial genital herpes (Centers for Disease Control and Prevention** 2022)	**Recurrent herpes labialis (Cohen** 2019)	**Recurrent genital herpes (Centers for Disease Control and Prevention** 2022)
Acyclovir 400 mg orally three times daily for 7–10 days or 200 mg orally 5 times a day for 7–10 days	Acyclovir 400 mg orally three times a day for 7–10 days	Acyclovir 200-400 mg orally 5 times a day for 5 days	Acyclovir 800 mg three times orally for 2 days or 800 mg orally twice daily for 5 days
	Famciclovir 250 mg orally three times a day for 7–10 days	Famciclovir 1500mg orally daily for one day	Famciclovir 1000mg orally twice daily for one day
	Valacyclovir 1000 mg orally twice daily for 10 days	Valacyclovir 2000 mg orally 12hourly for a day	Valacyclovir 500 mg orally twice daily for 3 days

- Topical antiviral agents such as 5% acyclovir cream/ointment and 1% penciclovir cream can also be used for episodic treatment of herpes labialis.

- Daily suppressive treatment can be administered if needed for frequent genital herpes. Antiviral suppressive therapy when administered to patients with frequent recurrences can reduce the genital herpes recurrence rates by 70–80% (Centers for Disease Control and Prevention 2022).

- Acyclovir 400 mg orally twice daily, valacyclovir 1000 mg orally daily, famciclovir 250 mg orally twice daily are among the regimens used for suppression. Valacyclovir 500 mg orally daily can also be used but is less effective than other regimens if episodes are $\geq$ 10/year (Centers for Disease Control and Prevention 2022)

- Periodic assessment to see if the suppressive treatment needs to be continued or not should be done as the frequency of relapses tends to decrease with time.

- **Inoculation herpes simplex**: This can occur at any part of the body if there is inoculation of HSV in that area (Fig. 6.8). Therefore, always rule out inoculation herpes in cases where there are localized cluster of vesicles.

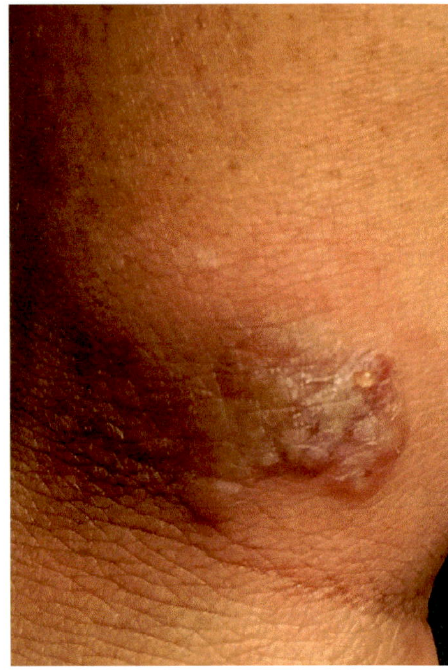

Fig. 6.8 Inoculation herpes on the wrist

6.9 Herpes Zoster (HZ)

- Herpes zoster, commonly called as Shingles, is caused by varicella zoster virus. It occurs in those individuals who had chicken pox in the past. After chicken pox subsides, the virus resides in the neurons in a dormant state. It manifests as HZ when it gets activated.

- Risk of HZ significantly increases in adults who are 50 years and older (John and Canaday 2017).

- However, HZ can occur at any age including children (Yellumahanthi 2004).

- HZ clinically manifests as painful blistering rash involving a single dermatome (Fig. 6.9). It is always unilateral and does not cross the midline of the body. The vesicles are arranged in several clusters. The lesions start as maculopapular lesions and then transform into vesicles. It takes about 2–4 weeks for the lesions to heal (John and Canaday 2017).

- Often the rash is preceded by symptoms such as pain or tingling or numbness confined to the affected dermatome. These symptoms can occur few hours to several days prior to the onset of the rash (Jianbo et al. 2018).

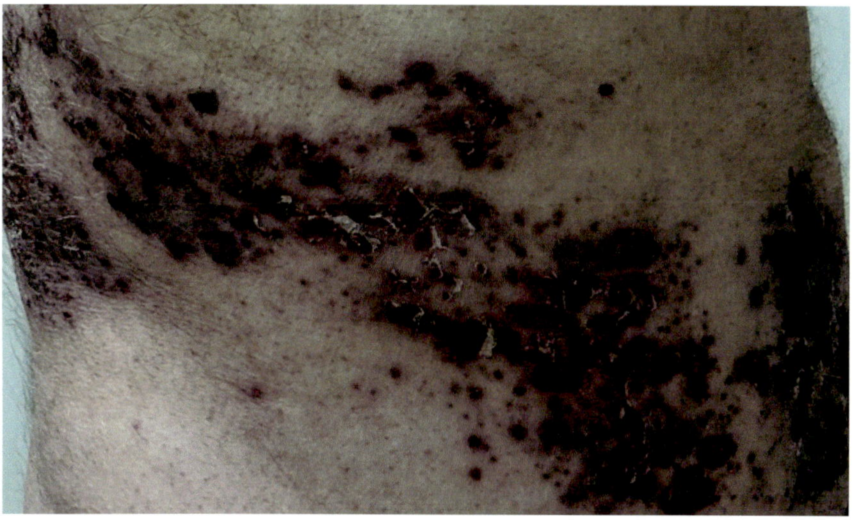

Fig. 6.9 Herpes zoster

- At times, this presence of prodromal pain without rash can pose diagnostic challenges when it occurs in those areas where life-threatening conditions can cause pain such as myocardial infarction when it occurs on the left side of the chest or appendicitis when occurs near the right lower quadrant of the abdomen.

- Uncommonly, shingles can manifest only as pain along a dermatome without the characteristic rash. This condition is called as *Zoster sine herpete.*

6.9.1 Diagnosis

- Diagnosis is not difficult when it occurs with its classical presentation. When it is not typical, the vesicular fluid can be sent for NAAT (PCR) testing (Jianbo et al. 2018).

6.9.2 Management

- Oral acyclovir, famciclovir and valacyclovir are all effective in treating symptoms of herpes zoster. Famciclovir is reported to be superior to valacyclovir in relieving the acute zoster pain (Ono et al. 2012).

- The efficacy of antivirals is best effective if administered within 72 hours of onset of the rash.

- Initiating antiviral treatment after 72 hours of onset of shingles may be recommended if new lesions are still occurring or if there are any complications such as neurologic or motor or ocular complications (Dworkin et al. 2007).

- Along with antiviral drugs, any analgesics such as NSAIDs can be given for pain relief if needed. In author's experience, most patients did not need anything more stronger than NSAIDs for pain control.

- Postherpetic neuralgia (PHN) is the most dreaded complication. Although there is no consensus on what qualifies as PHN, pain lasting for more than 90 days after the onset of the shingles is conventionally thought to be PHN (Watson 2011).

- If PHN occurs gabapentin, pregabalin and amitriptyline are among the oral drugs that can be tried. If PHN continues, a referral to dermatologist may help.

- The risk of having a second episode of HZ among immunocompetent people is estimated to be about 6.4% (John and Canaday 2017).

- Vaccine for shingles, shingrix can help in preventing shingles in those who were affected with chicken pox in the past.

6.10 Cutaneous HPV Infection (Verruca Vulgaris or Warts)

- Warts are benign growths that are caused by human papillomavirus (HPV).

- A common wart is less than 1 cm in size and is hyperkeratotic.

- Warts often have tiny black/red dots, that represent thrombosed capillaries on the surface (Fig. 6.10).

- Morphologically warts can be of different types. For instance, flat warts (Fig. 6.11) and filiform warts (Fig. 6.12). Filiform warts are finger-like hyperkeratotic growths.

- Based on the location, warts can be genital or extragenital.

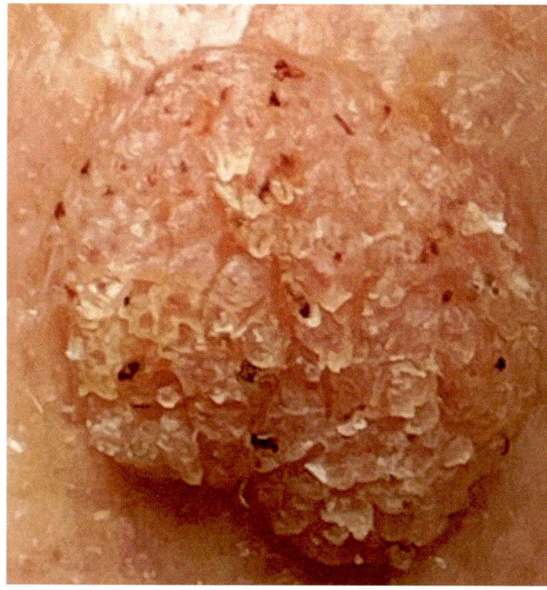

Fig. 6.10 Verruca vulgaris. Please note thrombosed capillaries

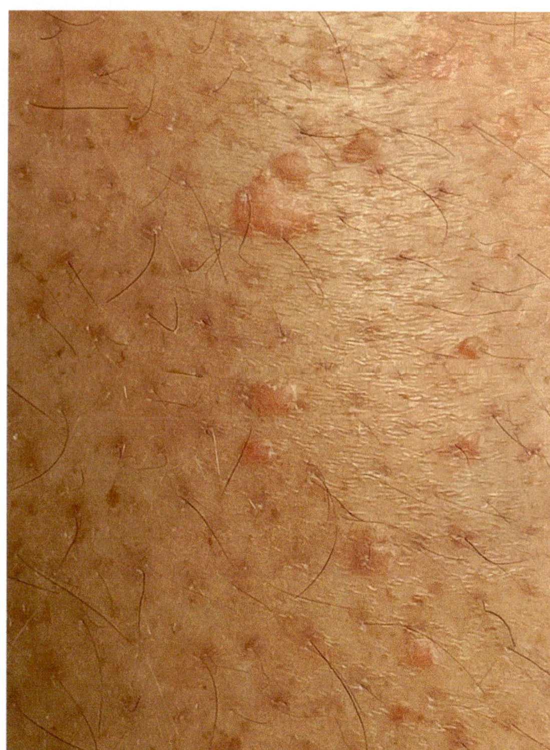

Fig. 6.11 Flat warts

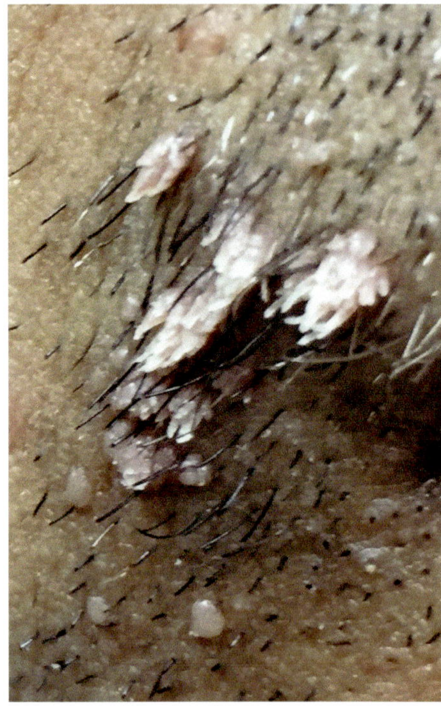

Fig. 6.12 Filiform warts (flat warts can also be seen)

6.10.1 Diagnosis

- Warts can usually be diagnosed clinically. The presence of thrombosed capillaries that is manifested as black or red dot to the naked eye, if present is helpful in diagnosis. Palmar and plantar warts can be differentiated from callosities by the fact that unlike callosities, they interfere with skin lines (dermatoglyphics). In adults, seborrheic keratosis, squamous cell cancer can sometimes come in the differential diagnosis of warts. Skin biopsy can be done for histopathological diagnosis if necessary for the confirmation of the clinical diagnosis of warts.

- Warts are self-limiting; most of them clearing within about two years in young people (Williams et al. 1993).

- In adults, it might persist for years if untreated (Sterling 2019).

6.10.2 Management

- Various regimens are used. None of these cures HPV. They mainly act by destruction or immunomodulation (Arndt 2011). Given below are some of the regimens given for extragenital warts:

- Daily application of salicylic acid. It is available as a maximum strength of 40% without prescription in the US.

- Cryotherapy is often the most common office-based treatment modality employed. The reported median cure rate for it is about 49%. Cryotherapy is done with liquid nitrogen with an approximate freeze time of 5–30 s (based on size and site of the lesion) is repeated every 2–3 weeks (Sterling et al. 2014).

- 5% 5-fluorouracil twice daily: The reported cure rate with occlusion for 4 weeks is about 95% in one study (Sterling et al. 2014).

- Imiquimod 5% cream is to be applied 3–5 times/week for a maximum of 16 weeks (Arndt et al. 2011).

- Tretinoin 0.1% cream or gel.

- Surgical excision can also be done.

- Genital warts: Specific treatment includes topical podophyllotoxin 0.5% solution for 3 days on and 4 days off for 4 weeks or sinecatechins (15% ointment). Cryotherapy can also be used.

- Please see Chap. 15, 'Feet' Figs. 15.6 and 15.7 for plantar wart and periungual wart pictures, respectively.

Fungal Infections

Dermatophytosis
Cutaneous Candidiasis.

6.11 Dermatophytosis (Ring Worm)

- It is a superficial fungal infection that affects the skin, hair and nails.

- It is caused by fungi known as dermatophytes. The causative species belong to genus Microsporum, Trichophyton and Epidermophyton (Kovitwanichkanont and Chong 2019).

- The name of the skin condition affected by them is often based on the part of the body that is involved—Tinea corporis (Body), Tinea capitis (Head), Tinea faciei (face), Tinea barbae (beard) Tinea cruris (body folds), Tinea manuum (hand), Tinea pedis (Feet), Tinea unguium (onychomycosis).

- **Clinical presentation**: The exact clinical presentation can vary depending on the body site involved.
  - The classical description of ringworm is annual erythematous plaques with central clearing and raised borders with fine scaling.
  - Tinea corporis (T. corporis) (Fig. 6.13), tinea barbae, tinea cruris, tinea faciei presents with classical description.

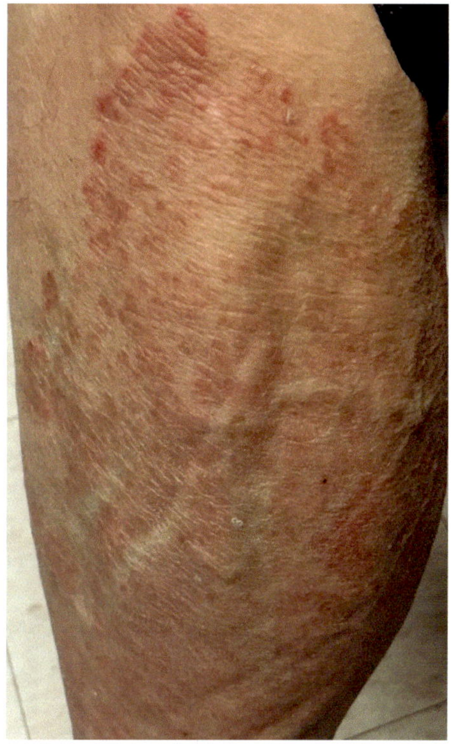

Fig. 6.13 Tinea corporis. Borders are raised

6.11.1 Tinea Manuum (T. manuum)

- It is the name given to dermatophytic infection that affects either dorum of the hands or palms or finger web spaces (Chamorro et al. 2024). The affected palms present with diffuse scaling of palms and the finger creases are usually accentuated (Craddock and Schieke 2019).

- The dorsa, if affected, has classical T. corporis presentation. Often only one hand is involved along with the involvement of both feet—giving it the name—'Two feet, one hand syndrome'.

6.11.2 Tinea Cruris (Jock Itch) (T. cruris)

- Is the name given if dermatophytic infection involves either groin or pubic area or genitalia or perianal or perineal region (Pippin et al. 2024).

- It manifests classically as erythematous annular plaques. When groin is involved, it usually spares the genitalia (Rippon 1988).

- Please see Chap. 13, 'Genitals and Groin' for the picture of T. cruris (Fig. 13.1) and details regarding its clinical manifestations, diagnosis and management.

6.11.3 *Tinea Pedis (T. pedis)*

- Dermatophytic infection of feet is termed tinea pedis.
- Can manifest as either interdigital or moccasin or bullous/vesicular form.
- Interdigital form can present with peeling or maceration or fissuring or scaling affecting the lateral toe clefts.
- Moccasin type presents as patchy or diffuse scaling on the soles and the lateral and medial aspects of the feet (Fig. 6.14).
- Bullous form manifests as blisters on the sole.
- Please see Chap. 15, 'Feet' section on tinea pedis for more details on its clinical presentation, diagnosis and management.

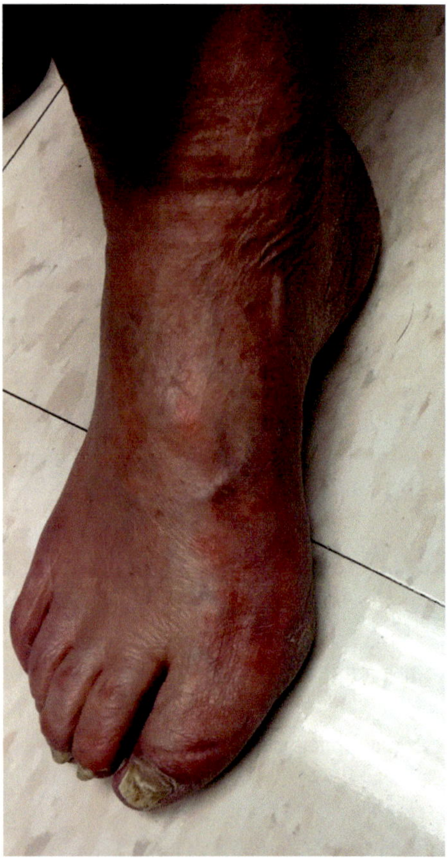

Fig. 6.14 Tinea pedis (moccasin distribution). Also note Tinea ungiuum

6.11.4 Tinea Capitis (T. capitis) (Figs. 6.15 and 6.16)

- Dermatophytic infection of the head is termed tinea capitis. It can be associated with both alopecia and scaling. Alopecia can be both scarring and non-scarring.

- Several variations of presentations are seen.

- If hair loss is present, it is usually patchy. In the non-scarring type of alopecia, the clinical picture can vary depending on the level of breakage of hair. For instance, if the hair is broken at the surface of the scalp, it manifests as patchy hair loss with 'Black dot' appearance. Otherwise, it can present as patchy alopecia with 'gray scales or patches' (Craddock and Schieke 2019; Bershow 2022).

- Sometimes, it can also present as diffuse scaling without alopecia (Bershow 2022).

- Favus (seen with yellow crusts) and kerion (present with boggy swelling) are the inflammatory types of T. capitis and that can result in scarring alopecia (Bershow 2022).

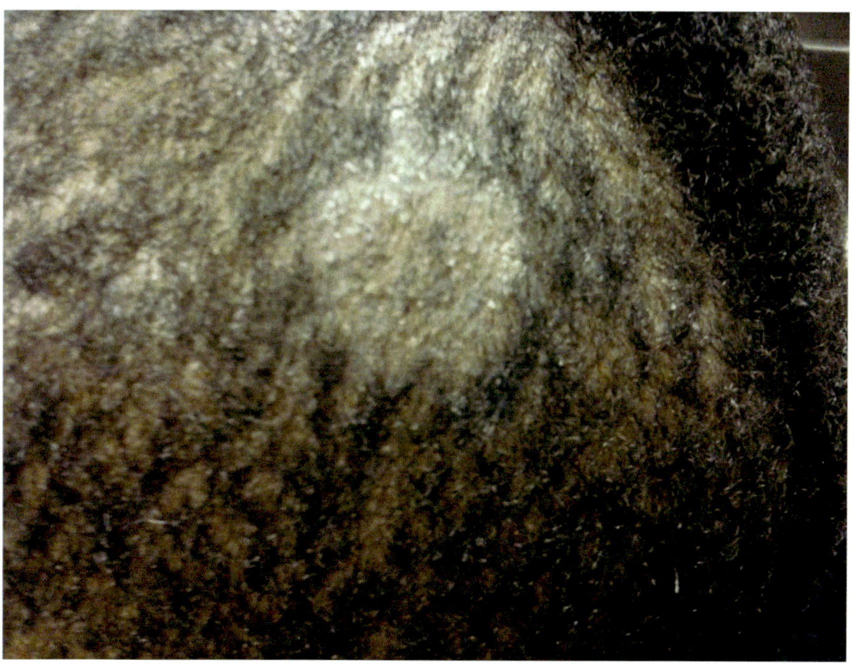

Fig. 6.15 T. capitis with non-cicatricial hair loss

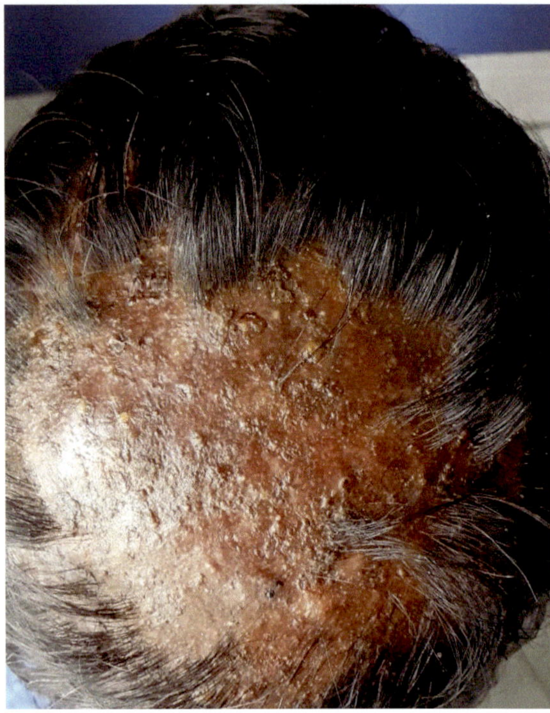

Fig. 6.16 T.capitis with cicatricial hair loss. *Courtesy* Dr. P.V. Krishna Rao, Dermatologist, India

6.11.5 Onychomycosis or Tinea Unguim or Nail Fungus

– Please see Chap. 16, 'Common Disorders Of Nails' for clinical presentation, diagnosis and management of onychomycosis.

6.11.6 Diagnosis of Dermatophytic Infections

– Skin scrapings can be scraped and examined under potassium hydroxide (KOH) preparation.

– Scrapings can also be sent for fungal culture.

– Skin biopsy can be done for histopathological examination.

– For T. capitis, culture is preferred. It is best to initiate treatment while waiting on culture results as culture often takes few weeks to report.

6.11.7 Management of Dermatophytes

- **T. capitis**: Only topical treatment has no role. Griseofulvin is usually the preferred choice. Oral terbinafine is another option. Fluconazole and itraconazole can also be used although they are not FDA approved for this condition. This can be supplemented with shampoos such as selenium sulfide shampoos (Information for Healthcare Professionals 2020).

- **T. corporis/cruris/manuum/pedis**: Topical allylaamines (Terbinafine) and imidazoles such as ketoconazole, clotrimazole or any other newer topical anti-fungals can be used. Oral antifungal therapy such as terbinafine 250 mg/day for 2–8 weeks [42] or fluconazole 150 mg/week for 4 weeks (Craddock and Schieke 2019) can be administered in adult cases not responding to topical antifungals or for extensive lesions.

6.12 Cutaneous Candidiasis

- Candidia albicans is the common organism causing it (Taudorf et al. 2019).

- It is an opportunistic infection.

- Affects mainly intertriginous areas.

- Besides pruritus, there could be tenderness, and pain in the affected areas.

- Typical Distribution: Inframammary, axillae, groins, perineal and intergluteal cleft.

- Manifests as moist looking, well-demarcated, erythematous patches (Fig. 6.17).

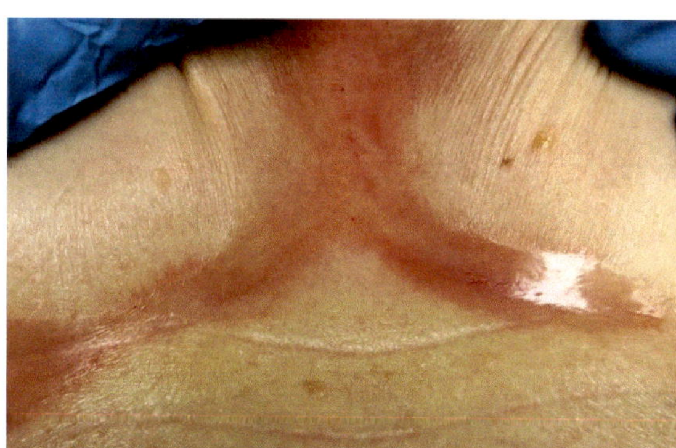

Fig. 6.17 Inframammary candidiasis

6.12.1 Diagnosis

- Diagnosis is based on clinical findings confirmed with direct microscopy with KOH or culture (Taudorf et al. 2019). Direct microscopy with KOH preparation visualizes pseudohyphae and yeast forms.

6.12.2 Management

- Topical antifungals: Nystatin, imidazole or azole cream or powder can be used (Taudorf et al. 2019).

- Oral antifungals: Fluconazole is a common drug that is used if refractory to topical agents or lesions are wide spread.

- Prevention: Keep intertriginous areas dry and regular use of antifungal powder.

Miscellaneous

6.13 Scabies

- Caused by mite, Sarcoptes scabiei.
- Classical presentation is with papulovesicular lesions.
- Incubation period is 4–8 weeks (CDC—Scabies—Resources for Health Professionals—Medications 2019).
- Common sites of involvement are finger webs, back of elbows, anterior axillary fold, areola and nipples, inner sides of thighs and male genitalia. In any given patient, all these sites need not have to be involved.
- Intense itching is present.
- Itching could be more in the nights. Therefore, a history of if itching that is more in the night (or not) should be sought from the patient. If the itching is more in the night that can strengthen the suspicion of scabies.
- Scabies could also manifest as only nocturnal itching without any skin lesions.
- Usually history of affected family members or close contacts is present. Absence of such history does not rule out scabies.
- Pathognomonic lesion is a burrow.
- Burrows are formed as a result of female mite tunneling immediately beneath the skin surface. Burrows appear as skin-colored lines or serpiginous grayish-white lines. They are common in finger webs, front of the wrist, back of the elbow. (Prevention and for DC and CDC—Scabies—General Information—Frequently Asked Questions (FAQs) 2020).

6.13.1 Diagnosis

- Demonstration of mites or feces or eggs by light microscopy, dermoscopy or any other high-resolution imaging method confirms definitive diagnosis of scabies (Sunderkötter et al. 2021).

- A clinical diagnosis of scabies can be made if there is a suspicion and other diagnoses cannot explain for the patient's clinical presentation.

- To make a clinical diagnosis of scabies, a known contact does not need to be present always. History of affected family members need not have to be present always.

- Please do not confine yourself to classical textbook presentation to diagnose scabies as scabies is known to be a great mimicker.

- Given that scabies can have various clinical presentations, recommend having a high suspicion for scabies in any patient with papulovesicular lesions and thus have a low threshold to treat for scabies in such population.

6.13.2 Treatment

- Treating patient's contacts and those living in the household is a part of scabies management. Advice regarding how to disinfect the clothing and other items at home needs to be provided.

- Topical 5% permethrin is the commonly prescribed drug. It can be used for anybody older than 2 months. Patients need to be instructed to apply the medicine from neck to toes and wait at least 8–12 hours before washing it (Sunderkötter et al. 2021).

- Crotamiton 10% lotion or cream can also be used for adults. In patients who did not respond to topical therapy, oral ivermectin in doses of 200 mcg/kg/dose can be used. The dose is to be repeated after one week (CDC 2019).

- Both patient and all contacts are advised to get treated on the same day.

Bibliography

Arndt KA, Schalock PC, Jeffrey. Lippincott's primary care dermatology. 2011.

Aslanova M, Ali R, Zito PM. Herpetic gingivostomatitis. PubMed. Treasure Island: StatPearls Publishing; 2024. Available from https://www.ncbi.nlm.nih.gov/books/NBK526068.

Bershow A. Fungal infections. In: Soutor C, Hordinsky MK, editors. Clinical dermatology: diagnosis and management of common disorders, 2e. McGraw-Hill Education; 2022.

Blaise G, Nikkels AF, Hermanns-Lê T, Nikkels-Tassoudji N, Piérard GE. Corynebacterium-associated skin infections. Int J Dermatol. 2008;47(9):884–90.

Bystritsky RJ. Cellulitis. Infect Dis Clin North Am. 2021;35(1):49–60.

CDC— Scabies—Prevention & Control. Centers for Disease Control and Prevention. 2019. Available from https://www.cdc.gov/parasites/scabies/prevent.html.

CDC—Scabies—Resources for Health Professionals—Medications. 2019. Available from https://www.cdc.gov/parasites/scabies/health_professionals/meds.html.

Centers for Disease Control and Prevention. Herpes—STI treatment guidelines. www.cdc.gov. 2022. Available from https://www.cdc.gov/std/treatment-guidelines/herpes.htm.

Chamorro MJ, House SA. Tinea manuum. 2023 Aug 7. In: StatPearls. Treasure Island: StatPearls Publishing; 2024. PMID: 32644474.

Chen X, Anstey AV, Bugert JJ. Molluscum contagiosum virus infection. Lancet Infectious Dis. 2013;13(10):877–88. Available from https://www.sciencedirect.com/science/article/abs/pii/S1473309913701099.

Chiller K, Selkin BA, Murakawa GJ. Skin microflora and bacterial infections of the skin. J Investigative Dermatol Symp Proc. 2001;6(3):170–4. Available from https://www.sciencedirect.com/science/article/pii/S0022202X15529011.

Craddock LN, Schieke SM. Superficial fungal infection. In: Kang S, Amagai M, Bruckner AL, Enk AH, Margolis DJ, McMichael AJ, Orringer JS, editors. Fitzpatrick's dermatology, 9e. McGraw-Hill Education; 2019.

Dworkin RH, Johnson RW, Breuer J, et al. Recommendations for the management of herpes zoster. Clin Infect Dis. 2007;44(Suppl 1):S1-26.

Fleming DT, Leone P, Esposito D, Heitman CK, Justus S, Chin S, et al. Herpes virus type 2 infection and genital symptoms in primary care patients. Sex Transm Dis. 2006;33(7):416–21.

Gao Y, Farah R. Acne, rosacea, and related disorders. In: Soutor C, Hordinsky MK, editors. Clinical dermatology: diagnosis and management of common disorders, 2e. McGraw-Hill Education; 2022.

Gawkrodger D, Ardern-Jones M. Bacterial infection—staphylococcal and streptococcal. In: Dermatology: an illustrated colour text. 6th ed. Elsevier; 2017. p. 50–1.

Gottlieb SL, Myskowski PL. Molluscum contagiosum. Int J Dermatol. 1994;33(7):453–61.

Haddock ES, Friedlander S. Poxvirus infections. In: Kang S, Amagai M, Bruckner AL, Enk AH, Margolis DJ, McMichael AJ, Orringer JS, editors. Fitzpatrick's dermatology, 9e. McGraw-Hill Education; 2019.

Cohen JI. Herpes simplex. In: Kang S, Amagai M, Bruckner AL, Enk AH, Margolis DJ, McMichael AJ, Orringer JS, editors. Fitzpatrick's dermatology, 9e. McGraw-Hill Education; 2019.

Holdiness MR. Management of cutaneous erythrasma. Drugs. 2002;62(8):1131–41.

Hordinsky MK, Soutor C. Clinical dermatology: diagnosis and management of common disorders. New York: McGraw-Hill; 2022.

Ibrahim F, Khan T, Pujalte GGA. Bacterial skin infections. Primary Care Clin Office Pract. 2015;42(4):485–99.

Information for Healthcare Professionals. 2020. Available from https://www.cdc.gov/fungal/diseases/ringworm/health-professionals.html.

Jianbo W, Koshy E, Mengting L, Kumar H. Epidemiology, treatment and prevention of herpes zoster: a comprehensive review. Indian J Dermatol Venereol Leprol. 2018.

John AR, Canaday DH. Herpes zoster in the older adult. Infect Dis Clin North Am. 2017;31(4):811–26. Available from https://www.ncbi.nlm.nih.gov/pmc/articles/PMC5724974/.

Johnston C, Magaret A, Selke S, Remington M, Corey L, Wald A. Herpes simplex virus viremia during primary genital infection. J Infect Dis. 2008;198(1):31–4.

Kovitwanichkanont T, Chong AH. Superficial fungal infections. Aust J Gen Pract. 2019;48(10):706–11.

Leung AKC, Barankin B. Herpes labialis: an update. Recent Patents Inflamm Allergy Drug Disc. 2017;11(2).

Leung AKC, Barankin B, Hon KLE. Molluscum contagiosum: an update. Recent Patents Inflamm Allergy Drug Disc. 2017;11(1).

Miller LS. Superficial cutaneous infections and pyodermas. In: Kang S, Amagai M, Bruckner AL, Enk AH, Margolis DJ, McMichael AJ, Orringer JS, editors. Fitzpatrick's dermatology, 9e. McGraw-Hill Education; 2019.

Moran GJ, Krishnadasan A, Gorwitz RJ, Fosheim GE, McDougal LK, Carey RB, et al. Methicillin-resistant *S. aureus* infections among patients in the emergency department. New Eng J Med. 2006;355(7):666–74. Available from https://doi.org/10.1056/NEJMoa055356.

Omarova S, Cannon A, Weiss W, Bruccoleri A, Puccio J. Genital herpes simplex virus-an updated review. Adv Pediatrics. 2022;69(1):149–62. Available from https://pubmed.ncbi.nlm.nih.gov/35985707/.

Ono F, Yasumoto S, Furumura M, Hamada T, Ishii N, Gyotoku T, et al. Comparison between famciclovir and valacyclovir for acute pain in adult Japanese immunocompetent patients with herpes zoster. J Dermatol. 2012;39(11):902–8. Available from https://www.ncbi.nlm.nih.gov/pubmed/22670895.

Pearson DR, J. Margolis D. Cellulitis and erysipelas. In: Kang S, Amagai M, Bruckner AL, Enk AH, Margolis DJ, McMichael AJ, Orringer JS, editors. Fitzpatrick's dermatology, 9e. McGraw-Hill Education.

Pippin MM, Madden ML, Das M. Tinea cruris. 2023 Aug 17. In: StatPearls. Treasure Island: StatPearls Publishing; 2024. PMID: 32119489.

Preda-Naumescu A, Elewski B, Mayo TT. Common cutaneous infections: patient presentation, clinical course, and treatment options. Med Clin North Am. 2021;105(4):783–97. Available from https://pubmed.ncbi.nlm.nih.gov/34059250/.

Prevention CC for DC and CDC—Scabies—General Information—Frequently Asked Questions (FAQs). www.cdc.gov. 2020. Available from https://www.cdc.gov/parasites/scabies/gen_info/faqs.html#:~:text=Tiny%20burrows%20sometimes%20are%20seen.

Rippon JW. Dermatophytosis and dermatomycosis. In: Rippon JW, editor. Medical mycology: pathogenic fungi and the pathogenic actinomycetes. Philadelphia, PA: Saunders; 1988. p. 169.

Sauerbrei A. Herpes genitalis: diagnosis, treatment and prevention. Geburtshilfe Frauenheilkd. 2016;76(12):1310–7.

Sterling JC, Gibbs S, Haque Hussain SS, Mohd Mustapa MF, Handfield-Jones SE, Hughes JR, et al. British association of dermatologists' guidelines for the management of cutaneous warts 2014. Br J Dermatol. 2014;171(4):696–712.

Sterling JC. Human papillomavirus infections. In: Kang S, Amagai M, Bruckner AL, Enk AH, Margolis DJ, McMichael AJ, Orringer JS, editors. Fitzpatrick's Dermatology, 9e. McGraw-Hill Education; 2019.

Stevens DL, Bisno AL, Chambers HF, Dellinger EP, Goldstein EJC, Gorbach SL, et al. Practice guidelines for the diagnosis and management of skin and soft tissue infections: 2014 update by the infectious diseases Society of America. Clin Infect Dis. 2014;59(2):e10–52. Available from https://academic.oup.com/cid/article/59/2/e10/2895845.

Sunderkötter C, Wohlrab J, Hamm H. Scabies: epidemiology, diagnosis, and treatment. Dtsch Arztebl Int. 2021;118(41):695–704. https://doi.org/10.3238/arztebl.m2021.0296. PMID: 34615594; PMCID: PMC8743988.

Taudorf EH, et al. Cutaneous candidiasis—an evidence-based review of topical and systemic treatments to inform clinical practice. J Euro Acad Dermatol Venereol JEADV. 2019;33(10):1863–73. https://doi.org/10.1111/jdv.15782.

van Lisette, Berger MY, Butler CC, Koning S. Interventions for cutaneous molluscum contagiosum. Cochrane Database Syst Rev. 2009;(4):CD004767–7.

Watson P. Postherpetic neuralgia. Am Fam Physician. 2011;84(6):690–2.

Williams HC, Pottier A, Strachan D. The descriptive epidemiology of warts in British schoolchildren. Br J Dermatol. 1993;128(5):504–11.

Yarom N, Buchner A, Dayan D. Herpes simplex virus infection: part I--Biology, clinical presentation and latency. PubMed. 2005;22(1):7–15, 84.

Yellumahanthi KDM. Herpes zoster in a 10 year old child. J Am Acad Dermatol. 2004;50(3):P111–1.

Chapter 7
Cutaneous Malignancy

Abstract This chapter provides an overview of the three types of common skin cancers: Basal Cell Carcinoma, Squamous Cell Carcinoma and Malignant Melanoma. The chapter discusses mainly from their clinical perspective. It provides details about the clinical presentation of various types of these cancers. It discusses the clinical features based on how one can diagnose these conditions. The chapter also discusses ways to diagnose them. It provides details of what type of skin cancers can be managed by the primary care providers and when they need to be referred to a dermatologist or a Mohs surgeon. For those skin cancers that can be managed in Primary Care, it provides details as to how to manage them. It also discusses the options available for those patients who are not surgical candidates.

Keywords Basal cell cancer (BCC) · Nodular BCC · Pigmented BCC · Superficial BCC · Squamous cell cancer (SCC) · Bowens disease · Keratoacanthoma · Melanoma · Malignant melanoma · Nodular melanoma · Superficial spreading melanoma · Lentigo maligna melanoma · Acral lentiginous melanoma

Skin cancer is the most common cancer in the US. One in five Americans will develop skin cancer in the course of their lifetime. The three most common types of skin cancer are

1. Basal cell carcinoma
2. Squamous cell carcinoma.
3. Melanoma.

7.1 Basal Cell Carcinoma (BCC)

– Is composed of cells similar to those in the basal layer of the epidermis and its appendages.

– It is the most common cancer of the skin.

D. K. Yellumahanthi, *Manual of Primary Care Dermatology*,
https://doi.org/10.1007/978-3-031-68406-7_7

- It is also the most common cancer in the US (Skin Cancer Foundation 2019).

- Risk factors: Although chronic sun exposure is a risk factor, intense and intermittent sun exposure (Kricker et al. 1995; Pelucchi et al. 2007) as identified by prior sunburns appears to have greater influence. Radiation therapy, immunosuppression, a fair complexion, red hair and a positive family history of BCC are among other risk factors (Kricker et al. 1995; Gallagher et al. 2020; Martinez et al. 2021; Robinson et al. 2013; Karagas et al. 1996).

- The four most common clinical types are:

  Nodular.
  Pigmented.
  Superficial.
  Morpheaform/Infiltrative.

7.1.1 Nodular BCC (Fig. 7.1)

- Nodular BCC constitute about 60–80% of BCC (Tanese 2019).

- Bleeding on slight injury is a common symptom.

- Appearance: Pearly white papule.

- Telengectases course through the lesion (Fig. 7.2).

- Erosion and ulceration could be seen.

- Although, erosion, ulcer and telengectasia can be seen, all of them may not be seen in every patient.

- Head and neck are the common areas (Firnhaber 2020) although it can occur anywhere.

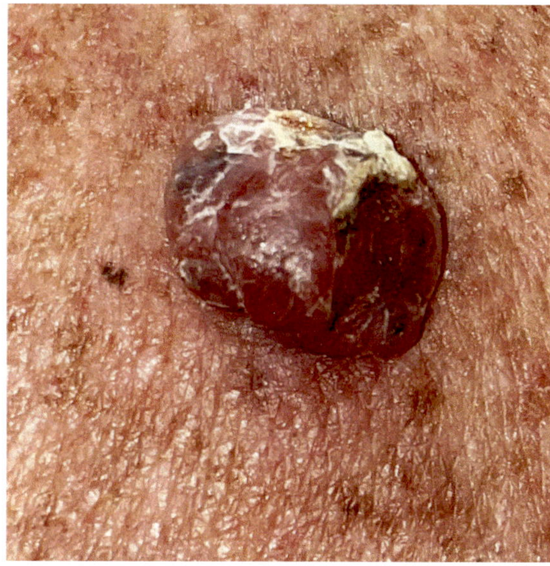

Fig. 7.1 Nodular BCC

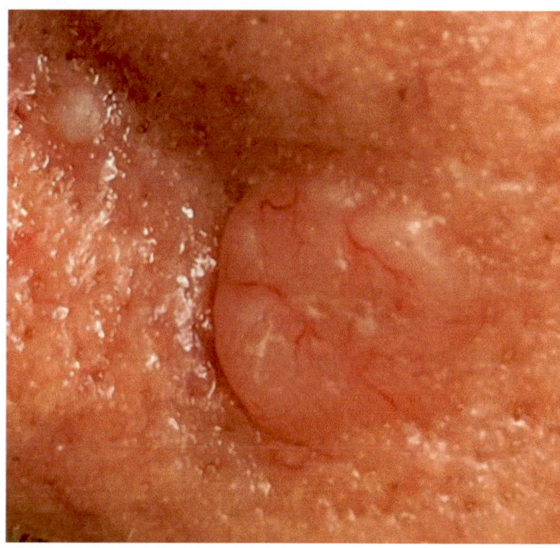

Fig. 7.2 BCC with telengectasia on the nose

7.1.2 Pigmented BCC (Fig. 7.3)

- Pigmented BCC is a broad term used for BCCs having pigmented features. It could be found in any subtype (Tanese 2019).
- This variety has all the features of nodular BCC, but in addition, brown or black pigmentation is present.
- Common in dark complexion persons.

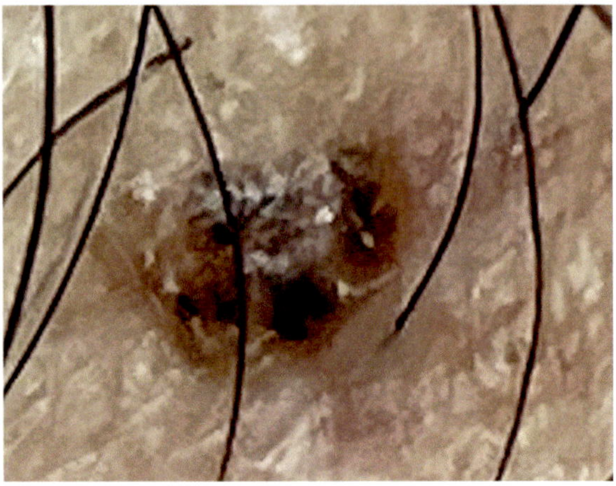

Fig. 7.3 Pigmented BCC

7.1.3 *Superficial BCC*

- It constitutes about 15% of the total BCCs. It is the second most common type of BCC (Fiessinger 2022).
- Common on the trunk and limbs (Scrivener et al. 2020).
- Frequently presents as a dry, psoriasis form, scaly lesion (Fig. 7.4). The lesions enlarge very slowly and may be misdiagnosed as patches of eczema or psoriasis.
- Edges of the lesion shows a threadlike raised border (https://www.pcds.org.uk/clinical-guidance/basal-cell-carcinoma-superficial#findings) (Fig. 7.5)—that is more conspicuous if the skin around the lesion is stretched.

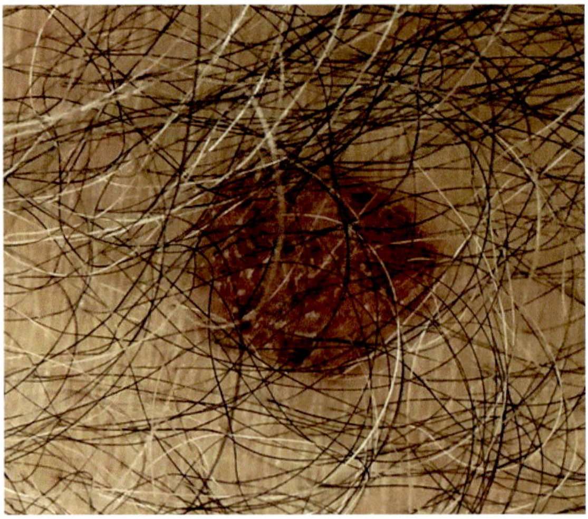

Fig. 7.4 Superficial BCC

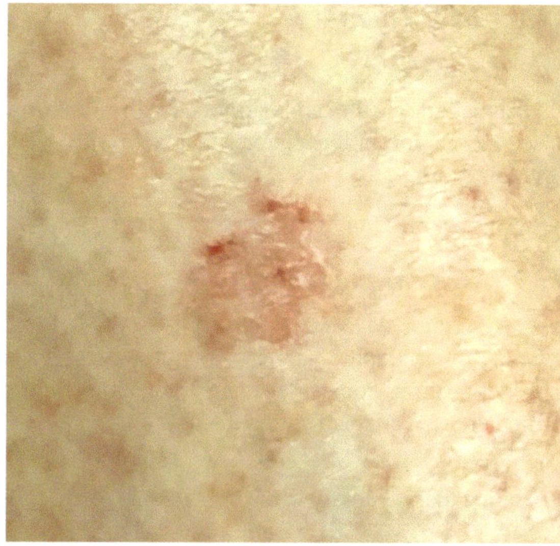

Fig. 7.5 Superficial BCC (Threadlike raised border at the edges)

7.1.4 Morpheaform/Infiltrative BCC

- Morpheaform BCCs constitute 5–10% of all BCCs (Tanese 2019).
- Often presents as a white sclerotic plaque.
- Most of these occur on the face and neck (Dourmishev et al. 2019).
- Margins are not well defined.

7.1.5 BCC Metastasis

- It has the least potential to spread from the primary tumor site.
- However, that does not mean that it should be taken lightly as a treatment in the advanced stage may need a large excision that can be disfiguring at times.
- Also, delaying the treatment can put the patient at the risk of having any specific functional impairment or mechanical discomfort.

7.1.6 BCC Diagnosis

- Histopathological examination is used for confirmation of the diagnosis. Please see the section in this chapter that states 'Diagnosis of Skin Cancer' for details on diagnosis.

7.1.7 BCC Management

- Mohs micrographic surgery, traditional surgical excision, curettage and electrodesiccation, topical agents, cryotherapy and radiotherapy are the various modalities available for treatment.

- Among these, surgery is the cornerstone of BCC treatment (Kim et al. 2018a).

- The assessment of risk for lesion recurrence is the most important step in the choice of treatment for BCC. Please refer to National Comprehensive Cancer Network guidelines at nccn.org to see if your patient's BCC falls under low risk or high risk recurrence.

- High risk for recurrence: Includes lesions on head, face, neck, genitalia, hands, feet, more than 2 cm lesion on trunk and extremities, any recurrent tumor, poorly defined borders, immunocompromised individual, morpheiform, perineural invasion (Schmults et al. 2023). This is not exhaustive list and please refer to National Comprehensive Cancer Network guidelines at nccn.org for complete list.

- High risk recurrence lesions need to be referred to either a Mohs surgeon or any other surgeon (or plastic surgeon) for wide local excision if a Mohs surgeon is not available.

- Low risk recurrence lesion: Includes features such as less than 2 cm in size on extremities and trunk. (Not including hands, feet, pretibial and genitalia), nodular or superficial BCC, well defined, primary lesion and immunocompetent patient (National Comprehensive Cancer Network (NCCN) 2021).

- Please refer to National Comprehensive Cancer Network guidelines at nccn.org to see if your patient's BCC falls under low risk or high risk recurrence.

- If it is a low risk recurrence lesion, it can be excised in primary care office with a surgical margin of 4 mm (Fig. 7.6) (Kim et al. 2018a).

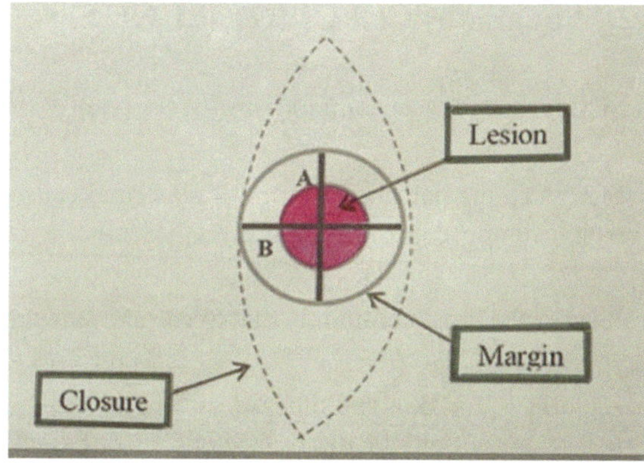

Fig. 7.6 Illustration of wide local excision

- In low risk recurrent BCC, if surgery is not feasible, the options include cryosurgery, topical therapy, photodynamic therapy and radiation therapy.
- Topical therapy is with imiquimod 5% cream and 5 fluorouracil (5FU).
- Imiquimod 5% is the favored topical treatment for BCC.
- 5% 5-FU with imiquimod 5% and PDT (methylaminolevulinate) in superficial BCC demonstrated that topical 5-FU is inferior to imiquimod and non-inferior to PDT (methylaminolevulinate) in the treatment of superficial BCC after 3 and 5 years of follow up (Peris et al. 2023).
- The efficacy of imiquimod compared with surgery for low risk BCC showed a successful response at 5 years, 82.5% for imiquimod vs. 97.7% for surgery confirming that imiquimod represents a good alternative to surgery for the treatment of low risk BCC (Williams et al. 2017). Side effects could include myalgia, headache and flu-like symptoms (Kulp et al. 2010).
- Cryotherapy: Studies showed that recurrence rates for cryothearpy range between 6.3% at 1 year to 39% after 2 years of follow up (Kim et al. 2018a).
- For cryotherapy, the cryogen used is liquid nitrogen and is used in the form of spray.
- Depending on the tumor thickness and type of BCC, the duration of freezing varies between 40–90 s. The ice ball needs to spread beyond the tumor by about 3–10 mm. Two freeze cycles are done usually (Collins et al. 2019).
- Pain, alopecia, blistering, pigmentation changes are among the possible side effects with cryotherapy (Collins et al. 2019).

7.2 Squamous Cell Cancer (SCC) (Figs. 7.7 and 7.8)

- SCC is second most common form of skin cancer (Skin Cancer Foundation 2019).

- SCC is an uncontrolled growth of abnormal cells arising in the squamous cells, which compose most of the skin's epidermis.

- It is caused most commonly due to chronic sun exposure.

- Light hair, fair skin and blue, green or gray eyes are among those at the highest risk of developing the disease (Skin Cancer Foundation 2019).

- Immunosuppression and usage of indoor tanning beds is also a risk factor for SCC (Skin Cancer Foundation 2019).

- Classical manifestation is a solitary scaly lesion located in a sun exposed area (Waldman and Schmults 2019).

- In about 4 to 6% of cases it can spread and can become fatal if untreated (Tisack et al. 2021).

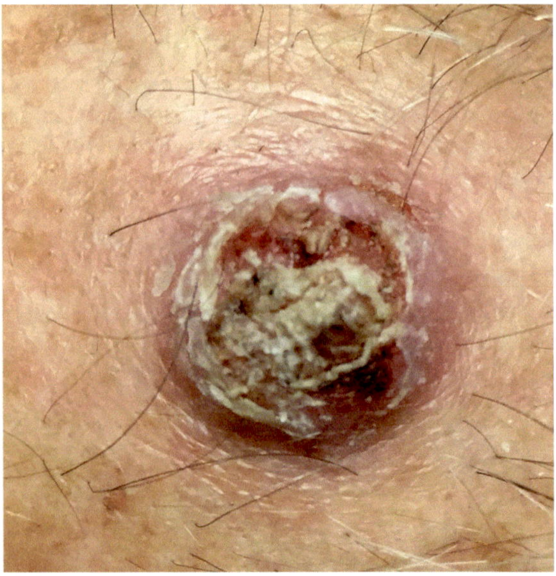

Fig. 7.7 SCC on scalp

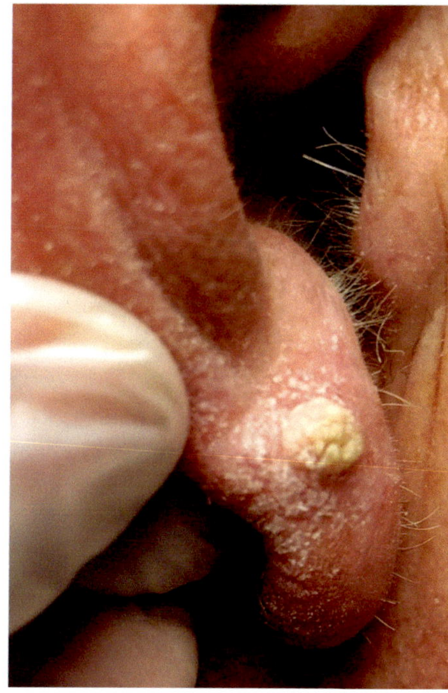

Fig. 7.8 SCC on external ear

7.2.1 Keratoacanthoma (KA)

- The status of keratoacanthoma is controversial. Some say that it is a separate entity while some say that it is a variant of SCC (Kwiek and Schwartz 2016).

- It begins as a papule that subsequently enlarges rapidly and when fully developed looks like a hemispheric or dome-shaped, skin colored nodule in which there is a smooth cracker filled with a central keratin plug (Kwiek and Schwartz 2016) (Fig. 7.9).

- After the rapid growing phase, it has a plateau phase and then involutes. Overall it may range between 4–6 months from when it began to when it involuted. It heals with or without significant scarring (Tisack et al. 2021).

- Occurs mostly on sun exposed skin.

- **Management:** Histopathological differentiation between KA and a well-differentiated cutaneous SCC (cSCC) can be difficult due to subtle distinguishing features. Therefore, although a traditional KA has a self-involution process, the current standard management for KA is similar to that of a well-differentiated cSCC, which is excision with a surgical margin (Tisack et al. 2021).

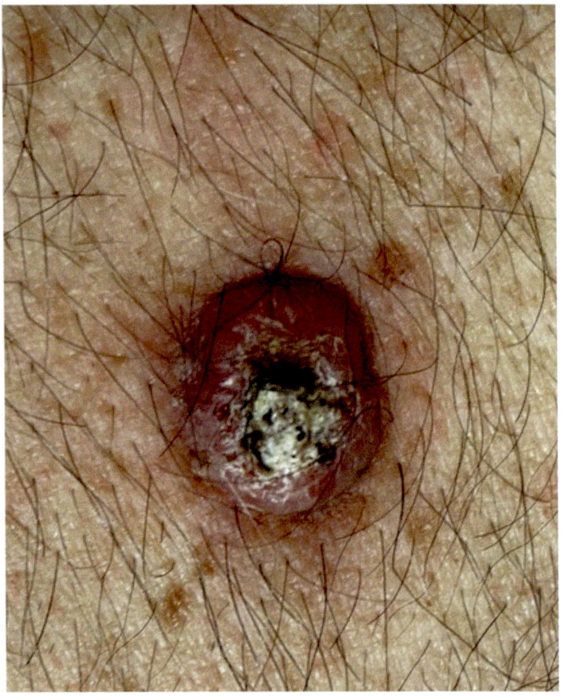

Fig. 7.9 Keratoacanthoma

7.2.2 Bowen's Disease

- Bowen's disease is in situ SCC of epidermis (Palaniappan and Karthikeyan 2022).
- May be found on any part of the body.
- Manifests as an erythematous, slightly scaly lesion (macule/patch) from a few millimeters to many centimeters in diameter. The lesion is sharply defined (Palaniappan and Karthikeyan 2022).
- Simple excision of small lesion is a reasonable treatment option.

Given the numerous presentations of SCC on the skin, there should be low threshold for biopsy of any suspicious keratotic, ulcerated or nodular lesions especially on the background of chronic sun exposure.

7.2.3 SCC Diagnosis

- Histopathological examination is used for confirmation of the diagnosis. Please see the section in this chapter that states "Diagnosis of Skin Cancer" for more details on diagnosis.

7.2.4 SCC Management

- Mohs micrographic surgery, traditional surgical excision, curettage and electrodesiccation, radiotherapy, cryotherapy and topical agents (In situ), are various modalities that can be used.

- Similar to BCC, the assessment of risk for lesion recurrence is the most important step in the choice of treatment for SCC. Please refer to National Comprehensive Cancer Network (NCCN) guidelines at nccn.org to see if patient's SCC falls under low risk or high risk recurrence.

- High risk recurrence lesions need to be referred to either a Mohs surgeon or any other surgeon (or plastic surgeon) if a Mohs surgeon is not available.

- Low risk SCCs, (The following list may not be exclusive. Please refer to NCCN guidelines at nccn.org for a comprehensive list) includes primary tumor, primary lesions <2 cm located on extremities or trunk (Not including hands, feet, pretibia and ankles), moderately or well defined tumor (National Comprehensive Cancer Network (NCCN) 2024).

- Low risk SCCs, can be managed in the primary care clinic by excision with 4 to 6 mm surgical margin (Fig. 7.6) (Kim et al. 2018b).

- Low risk SCC patients who are poor surgical candidates, radiation is an alternative (Kim et al. 2018b).

- Cryotherapy is an option for low risk SCC patients if surgery and other effective treatments are not feasible. For cryotherapy, the cryogen used is liquid nitrogen and is used in the form of spray.

- Depending on the tumor thickness and type of SCC, the duration of freezing varies between 40–90 seconds. The ice ball needs to spread beyond the tumor by about 3–10mm. Two freeze cycles are done usually (Collins et al. 2019).

– Role of topical treatment in management of cutaneous SCC in situ:

  For SCC in situ, the clearance rates with topical imiquimod is 57% to 80% (Love et al. 2009).

  Topical 5-fluorouracil clearance rates range from 54% to 85% with twice-daily application for 6 to 8 weeks (Bargman and Hochman 2003).

7.3 Melanoma

– Melanoma is a malignant tumor of melanocytes.

– Almost 80% will develop on previously normal-appearing skin (Primary Care Dermatology Society).

– Melanoma is caused by intense, occasional UV exposure more so in genetically predisposed individuals.

– The other risk factors include light complexion, light eyes, blond or red hair, heavy freckling, the occurrence of blistering sunburns in childhood, a tendency to sunburn easily and tan poorly. Family history of melanoma and presence of more than 50 benign nevi are also risk factors (Skin Cancer Foundation 2018; Saavedra et al. 2023).

– Most melanomas are black or brown in color. Melanoma also has various morphological/clinical presentations.

– Melanoma if not treated early, will result in death in 100% of the patients.

– There are four common types of melanoma

  1. Superficial spreading.
  2. Nodular.
  3. Lentigo maligna melanoma.
  4. Acral lentiginous.

7.3.1 Superficial Spreading Melanoma (Fig. 7.10)

- Most common type of melanoma (Pelucchi et al. 2007).

- It has no preference for sun damaged skin.

- Lesions may arise de novo or in association with the pre-existing nevus.

- ABCDE of melanoma can aid to diagnose it (Fig. 7.10).

  What are ABCDE of melanoma?

- Asymmetry: If the lesion is visually divided in to two equal halves in any direction, each half should look like mirror images of each other. If not, it is considered as asymmetry.

- Borders: If borders are not uniform it can be a suspicious sign.

- Color: In any given lesion, only one color needs to be present. If more than one color is seen, it can be a suspicious sign.

- Diameter: Usually lesions that are greater than 6 mm, need to be closely monitored.

- Evolving: Any recent change in size or shape or color or bleeding or crusting or any such changes need to be considered as suspicious signs.

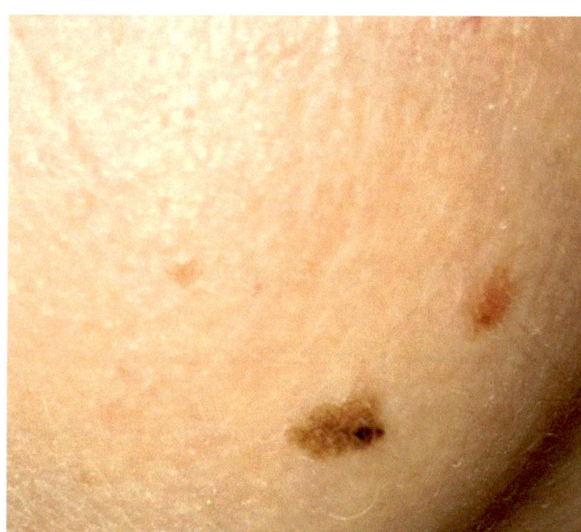

Fig. 7.10 Superficial spreading melanoma

7.3.2 Nodular Melanoma (Fig. 7.11)

- It constitutes to about 10–15% of all melanomas (The Skin Cancer Foundation 2018).
- It occurs primarily on sun exposed areas of the head neck and trunk.
- Could manifest as smooth and dome-shaped or polypoid or exophytic (The Skin Cancer Foundation 2018).
- These lesions arise without a clinically apparent radial growth phase.

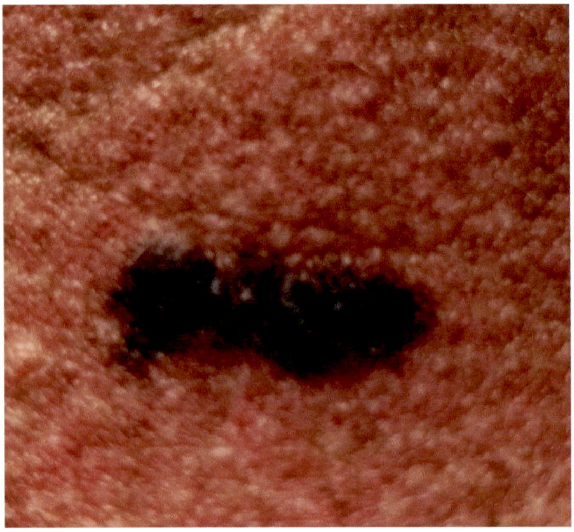

Fig. 7.11 Nodular melanoma

7.3.3 Lentigo Maligna Melanoma (LMM)

- More common in the older population.
- Cumulative sun exposure is important in the pathogenesis (Hassel et al. 2019).
- Most common on the face.

- Manifests as tan macule or patch that gradually progresses with varying shades. At this stage it is called as lentigo maligna (Fig. 7.12) (Hassel et al. 2019).

- After a radial growth period of several years, a vertical growth phase of invasive melanoma can develop. The lesion is then referred to as lentigo maligna melanoma (Fig. 7.13).

- A palpable area that is raised above the skin surface within the original macular (or patchy) lesion could mean that vertical growth occurred and the lesion transformed to LMM.

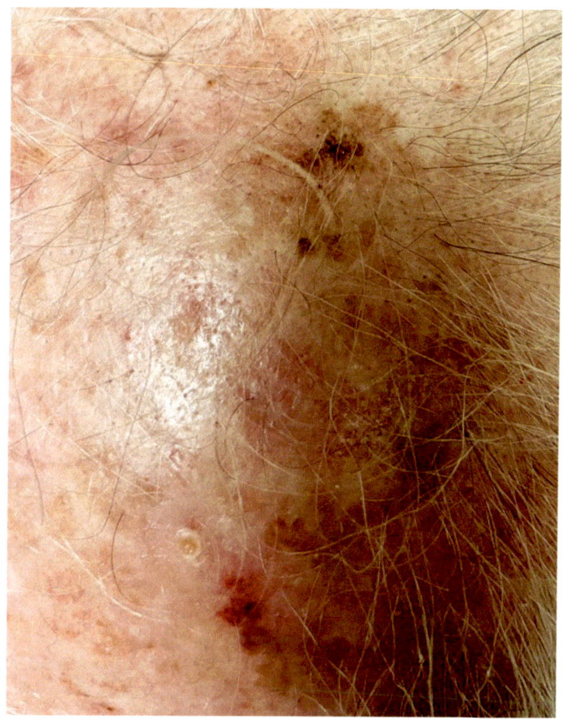

Fig. 7.12 Lentigo maligna on the scalp

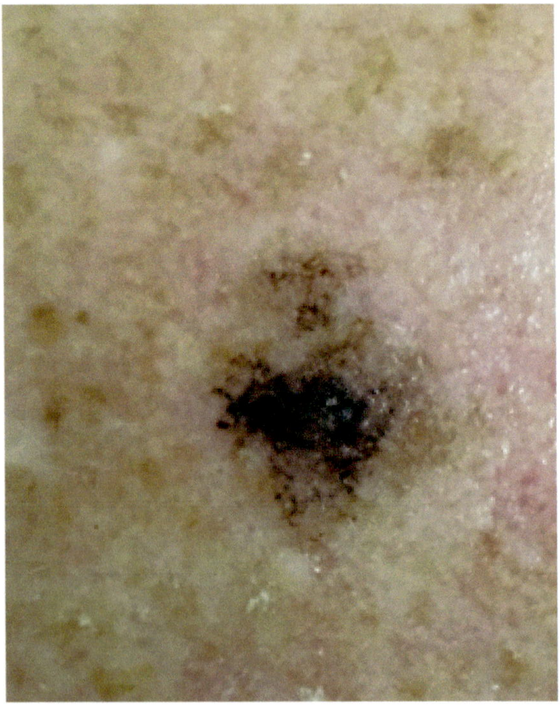

Fig. 7.13 Lentigo maligna melanoma

7.3.4 *Acral Lentiginous Melanoma*

- Most common type of melanoma in dark skinned and Asian populations (The Skin Cancer Foundation 2018).
- The median age is 65 years (Hassel et al. 2019).
- The most common site of melanoma in African Americans is the foot (Hassel et al. 2019).

7.3.5 *Amelanotic Melanoma*

- Differs from other melanomas by its lack of pigment.
- The lesion is pink erythematous, and could mimic basal cell carcinoma or granuloma pyogenicum.

7.3.6 *Melanoma—Metastasis*

- Early metastasis typically occurs through the lymphatics, and regional lymphadenopathy may be the first sign.
- Central nervous system (CNS) metastasis is the most common cause of death.
- The presence or absence of melanoma in regional lymph nodes is the single most important prognostic factor for melanoma.

7.3.7 *Melanoma Diagnosis*

- Histopathological examination is used for confirmation of the diagnosis. Please see the section in this chapter that states 'Diagnosis of Skin Cancer'.

7.3.8 *Treatment of Melanoma*

- Early excision remains the most important determinant of outcome.
- Recommend referral to a surgeon or a plastic surgeon to manage any melanoma cases.

7.4 Diagnosis of Skin Cancer

- The tools for diagnosis of skin cancer are thorough skin examination, dermoscopy and histopathological examination. Among these, histopathological examination provides definitive diagnosis.

7.4.1 *Skin Examination Tips*

- BCC, SCC and melanoma are to be ruled out based on history and morphology of lesions as described earlier in the chapter.
- In addition, from melanoma point of view, Ugly duckling sign can also come in handy.

- Ugly duckling sign: A pigmented lesion that looks different from other pigmented lesions on any individual should be approached with a high index of suspicion.

7.4.2 *Dermoscopy*

- It requires formal training using a dermatoscope. It is very useful and helps in diagnosing early melanomas and also helps in avoiding unnecessary biopsies. Recommend getting formal training in dermoscopy to all those who are keen on gaining expertise in skin cancer management. The details of dermoscopy are not provided here as that is beyond the scope of this book.

7.4.3 *Skin Biopsy/Histopathological Examination*

- The specimen for histopathological examination is provided through skin biopsy. Excisional biopsy is the standard type of biopsy for melanocytic lesions, if one wants to rule out melanoma. (There are some authors who say a deep shave biopsy (Saucerization) also may be sufficient) (Primary Care Dermatology Society).

- For ruling out BCC or SCC, either shave biopsy or punch biopsy or excisional biopsy can be done (The Skin Cancer Foundation 2018).

- Please see Chap. 18 "Skin biopsies and Cryosurgery" for details on various biopsy techniques.

7.5 Management of Skin Cancer—Prevention & Treatment

- Sun protection plays a key role in prevention of skin cancer.

- Avoid tanning and never use UV (ultraviolet) tanning beds.

- Cover up with clothing, a broad-brimmed hat and UV-blocking sunglasses.

- Use a water resistant broad-spectrum (UVA/UVB) sunscreen with an SPF of 30 or higher every day.

- Apply 1 oz (2 tablespoons) of sunscreen to your entire body 30 minutes before going outside. Reapply every 2 hours or immediately after swimming or excessive sweating (Skin Cancer Foundation 2022).

- Advice the patient to examine the skin head to toe every month. Scalp and nails also need to be examined carefully. Encourage them to see their physician every year for a professional skin exam.

- Management of BCC and SCC is as discussed earlier in the chapter.

- It may be appropriate for all patients with melanoma to be refered to a plastic surgeon or surgeon for further managment. Every patient with melanoma also needs to be referred to a dermatologist for periodic follow up.

7.6 Skin Cancer and Color of the Skin

- Skin cancer can also occur in people of color. In fact, studies show that African-Americans and other ethnic groups often have more advanced disease of melanoma at initial diagnosis and higher mortality rates than Caucasians.

- Therefore, people of color also need to be educated about skin cancer prevention.

Bibliography

Bargman H, Hochman J. Topical treatment of Bowen's disease with 5-fluorouracil. JCMS. 2003;7(2):101–5.

Collins A, Savas J, Doerfler L. Nonsurgical treatments for nonmelanoma skin cancer. Dermatol Clin. 2019;37(4):435–41.

Dourmishev L, Rusinova D, Botev I. Clinical variants, stages, and management of basal cell carcinoma. Indian Dermatol Online J [Internet]. 2013;4(1):12. Available from: https://www.ncbi.nlm.nih.gov/pmc/articles/PMC3573444/ [cited 2019 Mar 21].

Fiessinger LA. Nevi and melanoma. In: Soutor C, Hordinsky MK, eds. 12, 2nd ed. McGraw-Hill Education; 2022.

Firnhaber JM. Basal cell and cutaneous squamous cell carcinomas: diagnosis and treatment. Am Fam Physician. 2020;102(6):339–46.

Gallagher RP, Hill GB, Bajdik CD, Fincham S, Coldman AJ, McLean DI, et al. Sunlight exposure, pigmentary factors, and risk of nonmelanocytic skin cancer: I. Basal cell carcinoma. Arch Dermatol [Internet]. 1995;131(2):157–63. Available from: https://jamanetwork.com/journals/jamadermatology/article-abstract/5563651 [cited 2020 Feb 16].

Hassel JC, Enk AH. Melanoma. In: Kang S, Amagai M, Bruckner AL, Enk AH, Margolis DJ, McMichael AJ, et al., eds. Fitzpatrick's dermatology, 9th ed. McGraw-Hill Education; 2019.

https://www.pcds.org.uk/clinical-guidance/basal-cell-carcinoma-superficial#findings

Karagas MR, McDonald JA, Greendberg ER, Stukel TA, Weiss JE, Baron JA, et al. Risk of basal cell and squamous cell skin cancers after ionizing radiation therapy. JNCI J Natl Cancer Inst. 1996;88(24):1848–53.

Kim JYS, Kozlow JH, Mittal B, Moyer J, Olencki T, Rodgers P, et al. Guidelines of care for the management of basal cell carcinoma. J Am Acad Dermatol [Internet]. 2018;78(3):540–59. Available from: https://www.jaad.org/article/S0190-9622(17)32529-X/pdf

Kim JYS, Kozlow JH, Mittal B, Moyer J, Olenecki T, Rodgers P, et al. Guidelines of care for the management of cutaneous squamous cell carcinoma. J Am Acad Dermatol [Internet]. 2018;78(3):560–78. Available from: https://www.jaad.org/article/S0190-9622(17)32530-6/pdf

Kricker A, Armstrong BK, English DR, Heenan PJ. Does intermittent sun exposure cause basal cell carcinoma? A case–control study in Western Australia. Int J Cancer. 1995;60(4):489–94.

Kulp J, Levy S, Fein MC, Adams M, Furst J, Meng TC. Pharmacokinetics of imiquimod 3.75% cream applied daily for 3 weeks to actinic keratoses on the face and/or balding scalp. Arch Dermatol Res. 2010;302(7):539–44.

Kwiek B, Schwartz RA. Keratoacanthoma (KA): an update and review. J Am Acad Dermatol. 2016;74(6):1220–33.

Love WE, Bernhard JD, Bordeaux JS. Topical imiquimod or fluorouracil therapy for basal and squamous cell carcinoma. Arch Dermatol. 2009;145(12).

Martinez VD, Vucic EA, Becker-Santos DD, Gil L, Lam WL. Arsenic exposure and the induction of human cancers. J Toxicol [Internet]; 2011. Available from: https://www.ncbi.nlm.nih.gov/pmc/articles/PMC3235889/ [cited 2021 Apr 5].

National Comprehensive Cancer Network (NCCN). Clinical Practice Guidelines in Oncology: basal cell skin cancer. Version 2; 2021.

National Comprehensive Cancer Network (NCCN) Guidelines Version 1.2024 Squamous Cell Skin Cancer.

Palaniappan V, Karthikeyan K. Bowen's disease. Indian Dermatol Online J. 2022;13(2):177.

Pelucchi C, Di Landro A, Naldi L, La Vecchia C. Risk factors for histological types and anatomic sites of cutaneous basal-cell carcinoma: an Italian case-control study. J Investig Dermatol. 2007;127(4):935–44.

Peris K, Fargnoli MC, Kaufmann R, Arenberger P, Bastholt L, Seguin NB, et al. European consensus-based interdisciplinary guideline for diagnosis and treatment of basal cell carcinoma—update 2023. Eur J Cancer [Internet]. 2023;192:113254. Available from: https://www.sciencedirect.com/science/article/pii/S0959804923003568

Primary Care Dermatology Society. Melanoma—an overview [Internet]. Primary Care Dermatology Society. Available from: https://www.pcds.org.uk/clinical-guidance/melanoma-an-overview1

Robinson SN, Zens MS, Perry AE, Spencer SK, Duell EJ, Karagas MR. Photosensitizing agents and the risk of non-melanoma skin cancer: a population-based case-control study. J Investig Dermatol. 2013;133(8):1950–5.

Melanoma precursors and primary cutaneous melanoma. In: Saavedra AP, Roh EK, Mikailov A. eds. Fitzpatrick's color atlas and synopsis of clinical dermatology, 9th ed. McGraw-Hill Education; 2023. Accessed May 27, 2024.

Schmults CD, Blitzblau R, Aasi SZ, Alam M, Amini A, Bibee K, et al. Basal cell skin cancer, Version 2.2024, NCCN Clinical Practice Guidelines in Oncology. J Natl Compreh Cancer Netw. 2023;21(11):1181–203.

Scrivener Y, Grosshans E, Cribier B. Variations of basal cell carcinomas according to gender, age, location and histopathological subtype. Br J Dermatol [Internet]. 2002;147(1):41–7. Available from: https://www.ncbi.nlm.nih.gov/pubmed/12100183 [cited 2020 Feb 13].

Skin Cancer Foundation. Melanoma risk factors—The Skin Cancer Foundation [Internet]. The Skin Cancer Foundation; 2018. Available from: https://www.skincancer.org/skin-cancer-information/melanoma/melanoma-causes-and-risk-factors/

Skin Cancer Foundation. Basal cell carcinoma—The Skin Cancer Foundation [Internet]. The Skin Cancer Foundation; 2019. Available from: https://www.skincancer.org/skin-cancer-information/basal-cell-carcinoma/

Skin Cancer Foundation. Sunscreen—The Skin Cancer Foundation [Internet]. The Skin Cancer Foundation; 2022. Available from: https://www.skincancer.org/skin-cancer-prevention/sun-protection/sunscreen/

Tanese K. Diagnosis and management of basal cell carcinoma. Curr Treat Options Oncol. 2019;20(2).

The Skin Cancer Foundation. Melanoma—The Skin Cancer Foundation [Internet]. The Skin Cancer Foundation; 2018. Available from: https://www.skincancer.org/skin-cancer-information/melanoma/

Tisack A, Fotouhi A, Fidai C, Friedman BJ, Ozog D, Veenstra J. A clinical and biological review of keratoacanthoma. Br J Dermatol. 2021;185(3):487–98.

Waldman A, Schmults C. Cutaneous squamous cell carcinoma. Hematol Oncol Clin North Am. 2019;33(1):1–12.

Williams HC, Bath-Hextall F, Ozolins M, Armstrong SJ, Colver GB, Perkins W, et al. Surgery versus 5% imiquimod for nodular and superficial basal cell carcinoma: 5-year results of the SINS randomized controlled trial. J Investig Dermatol [Internet]. 2017;137(3):614–9. Available from: https://pubmed.ncbi.nlm.nih.gov/27932240/ [cited 2021 Sep 5].

Chapter 8
Scalp

Abstract This chapter provides an overview of the common dermatological conditions such as androgenic alopecia, alopecia areata, telogen effluvium that involves the scalp. The chapter discusses mainly from their clinical perspective. It provides details about the clinical presentation of these conditions and ways to diagnose them; where appropriate it provides clinical information regarding how to diagnose them clinically. It also discusses their treatment options and where appropriate the circumstances as to when the patients need to be referred to the dermatologist.

Keywords Androgenic alopecia · Alopecia areata · Telogen effluvium · Trichotillomania · Dandruff · Scalp psoriasis · Seborrheic dermatitis · Actinic keratosis · Contact dermatitis · Acne keloides

Hair loss and flaky scalp are the two common symptoms with which patients with scalp issues come to the office. The common causes for both those categories are listed below. Besides hair loss and flaky scalp, actinic keratosis, allergic contact dermatitis and acne keloids are other common conditions that can be seen on the scalp.

Hair Loss

Approach to scalp hair loss:

First make sure whether you are dealing with a scarring type of alopecia or non-scarring type of alopecia. In the scarring type of alopecia, hair follicles are not visible and the whole of the scalp looks like as though it is a glazed surface without any hair follicles. Normally if you are seeing a scarring type of alopecia it may be appropriate to refer to dermatology as the differential diagnosis can be exhaustive and may be beyond the purview of primary care discussion.

If the hair loss is non-scarring alopecia which means hair follicles are seen, then the following 4 common conditions need to be ruled out:

1. Androgenetic alopecia (AGA).
2. Alopecia areata (AA).

D. K. Yellumahanthi, *Manual of Primary Care Dermatology*,
https://doi.org/10.1007/978-3-031-68406-7_8

3. Telogen effluvium.
4. Trichotillomania.

8.1 Androgenetic Alopecia (AGA)

- Androgenetic alopecia (AGA) is the broad term given to both male pattern hair loss and female pattern hair loss. It is the most common form of alopecia worldwide, and is a result of an excessive response to androgens (Devjani et al. 2023).

- AGA in men manifests as gradual hair thinning that involves the crown and frontal areas of the scalp (Devjani et al. 2023).

- AGA in women is associated with diffuse hair loss and thinning that involves the frontal and vertex areas of the scalp (Devjani et al. 2023) (Fig. 8.1).

- While the hairline recession is commonly noted in males, the frontal hairline is maintained in females.

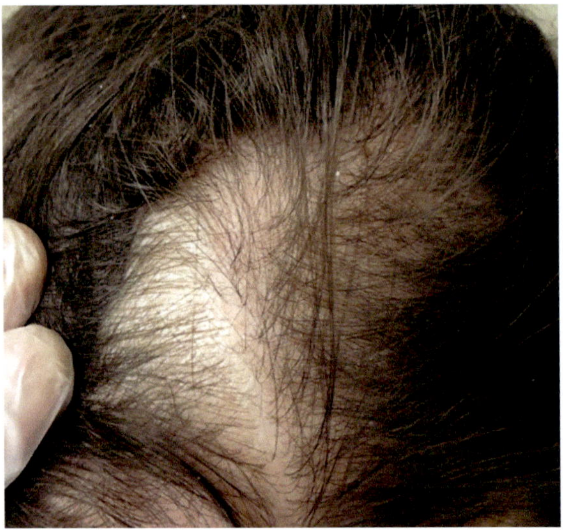

Fig. 8.1 Androgenic alopecia in a female patient

8.1.1 Diagnosis

- The diagnosis of AGA is usually done based on the history and physical examination. History needs to be sought in such a way that other common causes of hair loss such as telogen effluvium (TE) are ruled out. For instance, while the hair loss in AGA is gradual and insidious, the hair loss in TE tends to be more dramatic. Upon physical examination any signs of androgen excess (such as acne and seborrhea) needs to be ruled out. If present, needs work up to rule out any endocrinological causes for hair loss.

- Basic labs such as thyroid stimulating hormone (TSH), complete blood count (CBC), iron, ferritin and vitamin D testing can be done (Gordon et al. 2011) and addressed if found to be abnormal.

- AGA in males is quite obvious in diagnosis. In males, unless the history and physical examination indicate any underlying disorder or an associated disease, laboratory testing for the diagnosis of AGA is not necessary.

In females, AGA is subtle in presentation. Clues for diagnosis in females are:

- Patients with AGA usually complain about gradual reduction of hair density over a period of time. Sometimes noticeable day to day, hair loss may or may not be present.

- On examination, usually hair thinning is noted in the frontal, parietal or vertex region (Fig. 8.1), but diffuse thinning is possible as well. Often the frontal hair line is maintained.

- The hair pull test needs to be done in frontal, parietal, occipital and vertex regions. In AGA, the hair pull test could be positive in the frontal region, while it tends to be typically negative in the occipital region.

- To demonstrate hair pull test, about 50 hairs are grasped between the index, middle fingers and thumb from the base of the hairs near the scalp and firmly, but not forcefully, pulled away from the scalp. When the test is positive, more than 10% of the grasped hairs are pulled away from the scalp (Phillips et al. 2017).

- When in doubt, a scalp biopsy can be done to confirm the diagnosis.

8.1.2 Management

Men:

- Topical minoxidil 5% and oral finaseride 1 mg are the common treatments employed.

- Topical minoxidil 5% is applied twice daily. Shedding of hair initially, is an expected side effect of minoxidil use. Reassess after 6 months. Discontinuation of minoxidil usually results in shedding of hair within few months.

- Hypertrichosis, contact dermatitis and headaches are the common side effects (Devjani et al. 2023).

- Finasteride 1 mg orally daily can be used in those who are refractory to treatment with topical minoxidil or in whom topical minoxidil treatment is not feasible.

  It improves hair growth within one year of treatment, and further improvement can occur up to ten years of treatment (Rossi et al. 2011).

  Side effects include sexual dysfunction, erectile dysfunction, ejaculatory dysfunction and gynecomastia and these can resolve with cessation of the drug (Irwig 2012).

- Please note that oral Finasteride can lower the prostate specific antigen (PSA) levels.
  - For both the above drugs, treatment needs to be continued to sustain the results.

  - Hair transplantation is a therapeutic option for those patients with advanced disease.

Women:

- Topical minoxidil is commonly used. Both 2% and 5% topical minoxidil are effective in women (Olsen et al. 2002; Gupta and Foley 2015).

- Spironolactone is another common drug that is used in women with AGA. Doses from 25 mg orally daily to 200 mg daily have been used. This may be more effective in women who have excess androgen.

8.2 Alopecia Areata (AA)

- AA is the second most common cause of non-cicatricial alopecia.

- Alopecia areata is an autoimmune disease.

- It can coexist with other autoimmune disorders such as hashimoto thyroiditis and vitiligo.

- AA is the most common form of hair loss in children.

8.2.1 Clinical Features

- Often presents as single or multiple circumscribed patches of hair loss on scalp (Fig. 8.2). Sometimes other hairy areas such as beard, eyebrows can also be affected. Therefore, examination of those areas also needs to be done as it can help in the diagnosis and also in management.

- At the margin of the circumscribed patches sometimes noted are exclamation type of hair, which is basically hairs with distal part a little bit broader than proximal part.

- Nail changes: Pitting can be present.

- Given alopecia areata is an autoimmune condition, screening for other autoimmune conditions where appropriate needs to be done. In practice, commonly thyroid panel is done.

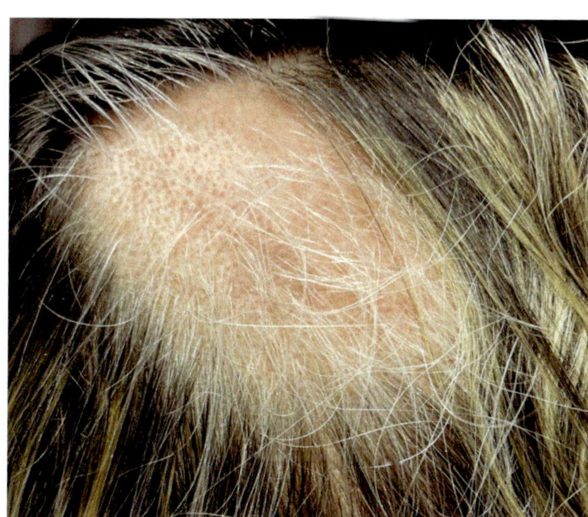

Fig. 8.2 Alopecia areata

8.2.2 Diagnosis

- Diagnosis often can be made clinically. Clinical manifestations, such as shape and appearance of the patches, exclamation point hairs and nail changes (pitting or sandpaper nails), can help in the diagnosis (Otberg and Shapiro 2019a).
  - In cases of doubt, a scalp punch biopsy can confirm the diagnosis of alopecia areata.

8.2.3 Management

- Alopecia areata has a variable course. While it is self-limiting in some patients, it could progress in others. Among patients with alopecia areata, about 5% develop hair loss of their entire scalp hair (alopecia areata totalis) and 1% may develop alopecia areata universalis (loss of total body hair) (Otberg and Shapiro 2019a).

- While limited involvement could have a favorable course, chronicity of the condition and involvement of nail, presence of other autoimmune conditions are among the poor prognostic factors (Alkhalifah 2011; Sterkens et al. 2021).

- All the drugs that are currently used for AA are only palliative and they do not alter the natural course of the disease.

- Topical steroids can be used for treatment of AA. Super potent topical steroids such as clobetasol propionate are more efficacious than less potent ones (Meah et al. 2020).

- Topical minoxidil can be effective and it can be prescribed along with any other topical or systemic agent.

- Intralesional corticosteroid injections are more effective than ultra(Super)potent/potent topical steroids.

- Triamcinolone 2.5–5 mg/ml is the common dose for scalp patches. While giving multiple injections, each can be up to 0.1 ml and about 1 cm apart. Maximum dose recommended in any given session is about 10–20 mg (Meah et al. 2020).

- Janus Kinase inhibitors (JAK Inhibitors): If more than 50% of the scalp is involved, patient might benefit from JAK inhibitors. Baricitinib was FDA approved for severe AA in adults. Ritlecitinib is approved for adults and children 12 years of age and older who have extensive hair loss (American Academy of Dermatology Association 2023).

– Systemic corticosteroids are also known to be effective in the treatment of alopecia areata.

– Although there are other immunosuppressive therapies that can be used for AA, it is best to refer to dermatologist if patients with AA are not improved with the above measures.

8.3 Telogen Effluvium

– Telogen effluvium (TE) is the most common cause of non-scarring diffuse hair loss (Grover and Khurana 2013).

– It is an acute or chronic diffuse hair loss that resulted due to increased shedding of telogen or resting hair.

– TE is acute, if duration is usually less than 6 months (Asghar et al. 2020).

– It is usually associated with a precipitating event such as any severe illness or stress, crash diet or certain medications, systemic conditions such as hypothyroidism, malnutrition, low zinc, low iron that are among many others.

– Hair loss typically manifests within 2–3 months after the precipitating factor (Asghar et al. 2020).

8.3.1 Diagnosis

– Diagnosis is usually based on history and clinical examination. Patients often describe losing lot of hair on a daily basis with routine activities such as combing, shampooing. They often bring shed hairs collected after shampooing or brushing during a certain period. After not shampooing the scalp hair for five days, if a wash test shows a count of more than 100 hairs that can be suspicious for TE (Asghar et al. 2020).

– The results of the hair pull test are diffusely positive in TE. When in doubt, scalp biopsy can be done to help with the diagnosis.

– A detailed history needs to be taken to try to identify any precipitation factors.

– The following labs can be done—complete blood count, ferritin, free T3, T4, thyroid stimulating hormone, anti-nuclear antibody, complete metabolic panel, sed rate, urine analysis to rule out any precipitating factors (Asghar et al. 2020).

– If clinically indicated, more relevant labs can be done.

8.3.2 *Management*

– Clinical course and prognosis of TE is variable. Normal hair regrowth can be expected within several months after the triggering cause is successfully identified and eliminated (Grover and Khurana 2013).

– Identification and subsequent management of trigger factors will be challenging if TE is of long duration.

– In the interim, treatment is usually supportive and assurance.

8.4 Trichotillomania

– Trichotillomania, is a type of hair loss that has manifested as a result of repetitive pulling of one's own hair.

– More common in children 10–13 years (Grant and Chamberlain 2016).

– The distribution of hair loss is quite peculiar, occurring in those areas that are easily accessible for pulling one's own hair. The areas of hair loss can be isolated or multiple. Scalp is the most common site (Grant and Chamberlain 2016).

– There could be some bruises and scratches in areas where there is hair loss (Recabar 2016).

– Often there is no history of self-pulling of hair as most patients are not aware of it (Grant and Chamberlain 2016).

8.4.1 *Diagnosis*

– Primarily clinical. Need to rule out other causes of patchy hair loss such as AA. Please see the section on AA in this chapter for details regarding how to diagnose AA.

8.4.2 *Management*

- Referral to psychiatry may be warranted. In early childhood, it is usually of short duration and could resolve spontaneously or with simple interventions. Management includes education of patient and/or parents.

- In older children and adults, there could be an underlying psychopathology and addressing it may be challenging (Recabar 2016).

Flaky Scalp

The common conditions that causes flaky scalp are

- Seborrheic Dermatitis.

- Psoriasis Scalp

8.5 Seborrheic Dermatitis (Fig. 8.3) (SD)

- Seborrheic dermatitis can occur in both children and adults. Usually does not cause hair loss.

- Lesions of seborrheic dermatitis have a greasy looking scale and erythema. Dandruff, which is the mildest form of SD is devoid of erythema and manifests as only flakes on scalp. SD is usually associated with pruritus.

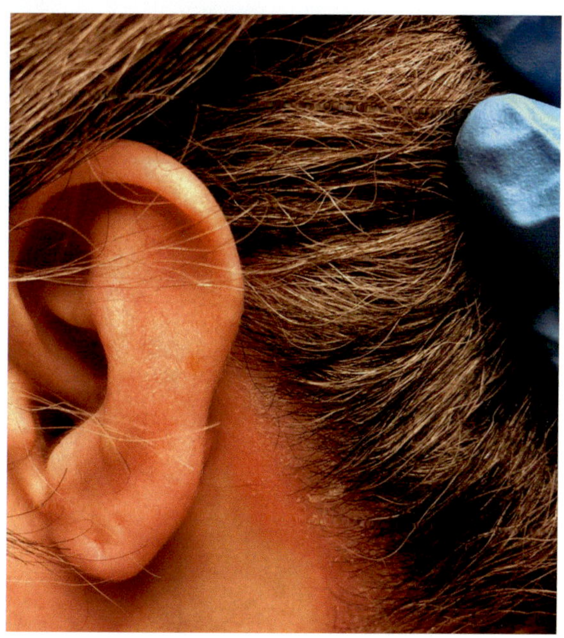

Fig. 8.3 Seborrheic dermatitis

- Along with involvement of the scalp, usually at least one of the other seborrheic areas like behind ears, glabella, nasolabial folds, front of the chest, pubic area is also involved.

- Therefore, in all cases of suspected seborrheic dermatitis, a total body skin examination is to be done with a more focused examination of seborrheic areas such as the eyebrows, glabella, nasolabial folds, beard area, retroauricular area, front of the chest and pubic area.

- Please see Chap. 5, 'Eczema' for more details on clinical manifestations, diagnosis and management of seborrheic dermatitis.

8.6 Psoriasis Scalp

- Can manifest as in isolation or as a part of psoriasis elsewhere.

- Manifests as erythematous plaques with adherent silvery scales (Fig. 8.4). Usually seen as an isolated plaque or multiple plaques with scales adherent to them. In between plaques normal scalp area without flakes is noted.

- Seborrheic dermatitis is the main differential diagnosis for isolated scalp psoriasis.

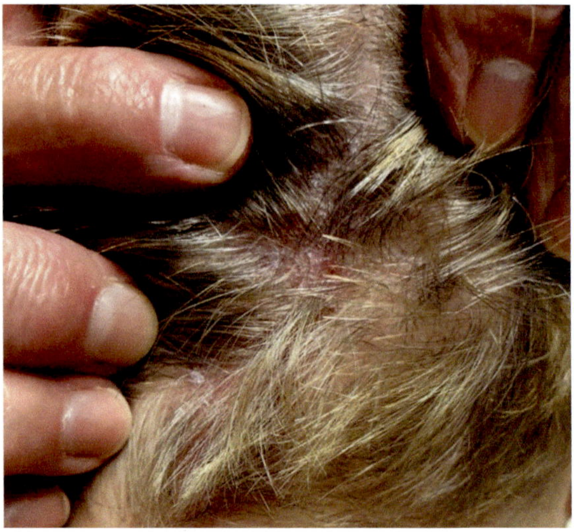

Fig. 8.4 Psoriasis scalp

- Psoriasis can be differentiated from seborrheic dermatitis based on the following:

  The presence of characteristic skin lesions elsewhere on the body—While the back of the elbows, sacrum region, front of knee are common sites for psoriasis, for seborrheic dermatitis, eyebrows, nasolabial folds, glabella, post auricular region, front of chest can be involved.

  Morphology of scales: Psoriasis manifests as silvery scales; seborrheic dermatitis as greasy looking scales.

8.6.1 Management

- There is no cure for psoriasis. It is usually chronic, with a history of waxing and waning.

- Patients are likely to have flare-ups if they discontinue therapy. The goal of therapy is symptomatic management.

- Tar or ketoconazole 2% shampoos and clobetasol propionate, 0.05% solution or lotion can be applied twice daily. Care should be taken not to over use the topical steroid. In author's opinion, it may be best not to prolong the use of steroid application for no more than 2 weeks at a stretch. It can be resumed after a gap of a week or two if needed. Calcipotriene scalp solution can be alternated with topical steroids.

- Systemic therapy may be warranted in cases not responding to above topical measures. Please see Chap. 3, 'Papulosqumous disorders' for details on systemic management of psoriasis.

- Refractory cases to topical medications can be referred to the dermatologist for further management.

Flaky Scalp & Hair Loss

- Both discoid lupus erythematosus (DLE) & tinea capitis (T. capitis), can cause both flaky scalp and hair loss. While DLE is usually more common in adults, T. capitis is more common in children. Also, the hair loss associated with DLE is usually cicatricial type (Fig. 8.5).

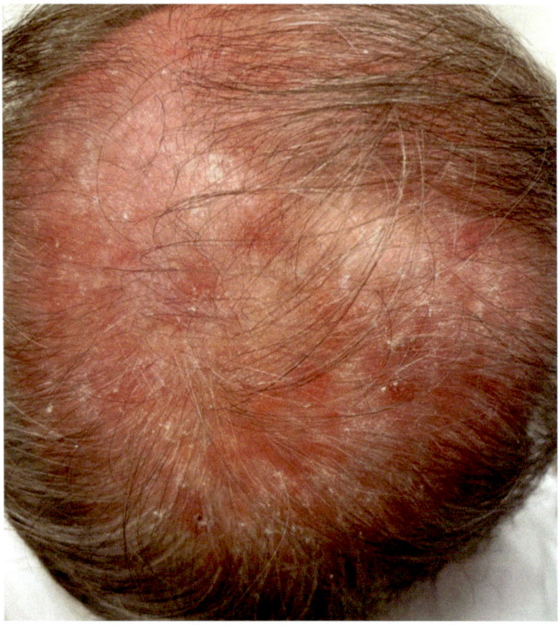

Fig. 8.5 Discoid lupus erythematosus with cicatricial alopecia

- T. capitis can cause both cicatricial and non cicatricial hair loss. Please see chapter 6, 'Common cutaneous infections' for details on clinical manifestations, diagnosis and management of tinea capitis.

  Please see Chap. 3, 'Papulosquamous disorders' for details on clinical features, diagnosis and management of DLE.

  Besides the above conditions, actinic keratosis and allergic contact dermatitis are also common causes of dermatitis on the scalp. Acne Keloidalis Nuchae is also an important condition in African Americans.

  Below is a brief clinically useful description of these conditions.

8.7 Actinic Keratoses

- Actinic keratoses (AK) are the most common epithelial precancerous lesions. They have the potential for malignant transformation to cutaneous squamous cell cancer (SCC). Therefore, treatment or close monitoring is recommended.

- AK are most commonly seen on chronically sun- exposed surfaces of the face, ears, balding scalp, dorsal hands and forearms.

- Commonly, they present as multiple, discrete, flat or elevated, scaly or keratotic lesions (Fig. 8.6).

- The lesions are usually relatively small, most being less than 6 mm.

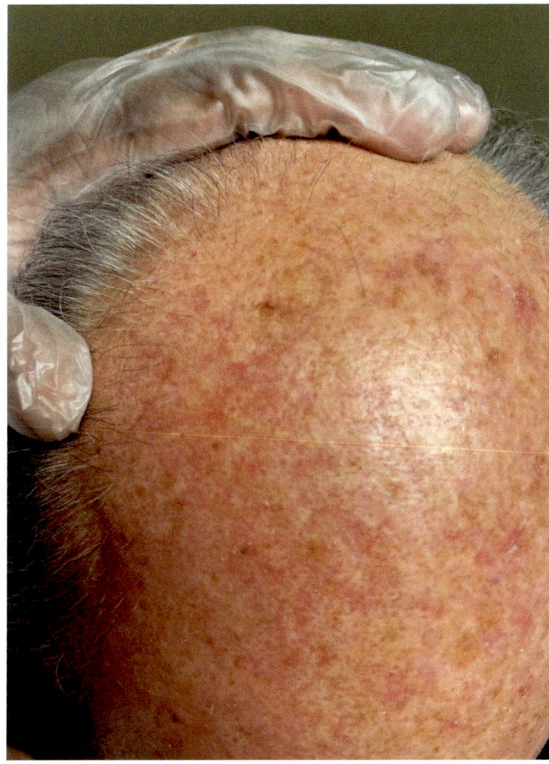

Fig. 8.6 Actinic keratosis

- Sometimes they are better felt than seen.

8.7.1 Diagnosis

- Diagnosis is made clinically. The classical clinical presentation is in the form of few minute scaly or hyperkeratotic lesions present on the sun exposed parts. Often there are signs of photodamage in the skin of the background.

- If the diagnosis is unclear, a skin biopsy can be done to confirm the diagnosis.

8.7.2 Management

- Cryotherapy with liquid nitrogen is effective and recommended way of treating AK when there are a limited number of lesions (Eisen et al. 2021).

- Although freeze time of 5–10 seconds with open spray technique is effective, a freeze time of more than 20 seconds is found to be more effective (Thai et al. 2004).

- A 1-mm to 2-mm freeze margin around the lesion is needed.

- Hypertrophic AKs need longer freeze times.

- For extensive, broad or numerous lesions, field therapy with either topical chemotherapy or photodynamic therapy (PDT) is recommended.

- Two agents most commonly used for topical chemotherapy are fluorouracil cream, 0.5–5%, or imiquimod 5% cream. Other agents approved are diclofenac 3% gel & tirbanibulin (Eisen et al. 2021).

  - Topical 5% fluorouracil (5FU) cream is the common agent used. Skin irritation is the most common side effect and patient needs to be educated about it at the time of prescribing the medication. Scaling, crusting, edema and flu like symptoms are other potential side effects with this medication.

  - It may be few weeks to months after stopping the 5 FU cream, patients will see the benefit of the medication. If any still persists, repeat treatment could be considered.

  - The ideal time to use 5% fluorouracil could be in the wintertime because while using this cream, patients should avoid being outside in the direct sunlight for prolonged periods of time.

- Imiquimod 5% cream: The recommended dose is to apply imiquimod 5% cream twice weekly for 16 weeks. It can cause irritation and erosions.

- Prevention of further sun damage is a key aspect of its management.

  Patients should be counseled regarding sun protection—Sunscreens with at least Sun protective factor (SPF) 30. Sunscreen needs to be reapplied every 2 hours or more frequently if there has been water exposure or excessive sweating.

  Also they need to be educated about avoiding sunlight during peak hours, usage of sun protective clothing and sun protective gear.

8.8 Contact Dermatitis

- Contact dermatitis is another important and common cause of dermatitis on scalp. Contact dermatitis of the scalp usually either manifests as a geographic pattern, for instance a band like pattern underlying a head band or **as** hairline pattern where rash is confined along the course of hairline and does not spread on to the scalp. The examples for former type are accessories such as headbands, hat, nickel hair pins and wig glues. Hair dye, perming solutions and hair gel are common causes of the latter type (Waldman and Grant-Kels 2021).

- Hair dye and topically applied medications are important causes of contact dermatitis on scalp.

8.8.1 Management

- Initial step is to eliminate the offending agent. Potent topical steroids such as betamethasone dipropionate 0.05% suspension are effective.

- If potential allergen is identified, advise the patient to avoid it. If allergen could not be identified, a referral to the dermatologist needs to be made for a possible patch testing and further management.

8.9 Acne Keloidalis Nuchae (Folliculitis Keloidalis Nuchae)

- Occurs most commonly in African American males.

- It usually occurs on the occipital scalp and nape of the neck.

- It begins as a chronic papular or pustular eruption (Fig. 8.7). Keloid formation may occur.

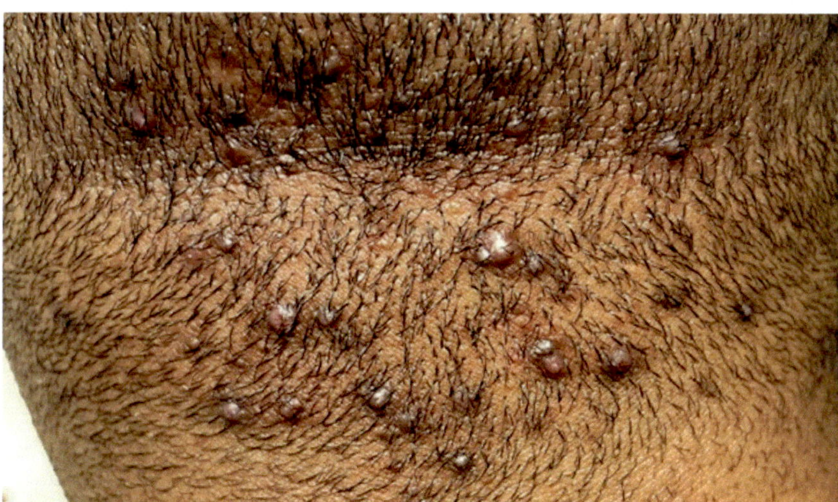

Fig. 8.7 Acne keloidalis nuchae

8.9.1 Management

- Intralesional triamcinolone in isolation or in combination with topical 2% clindamycin, or oral tetracyclines are usually the first treatment of choice (Whiting 2001; Otberg and Shapiro 2019b).
- Topical ultra(Super)potent or potent steroids with or without topical antibiotics can be used in mild cases (Otberg and Shapiro 2019b).
- The course is usually chronic and in recalcitrant cases need to be referred to a dermatologist.
- Please see Table 8.1 that summarizes common conditions causing flaky scalp, their key clinical features and management.
- Also please see Table 8.2 that summarizes common conditions causing hair loss, their key clinical features that aid in the diagnosis and their management.

Table 8.1 Common conditions causing flaky scalp: key clinical features and management

Common skin diseases that cause flaky scalp	Key clinical features	Management
Dandruff	- Confined only to the scalp. No erythema. Flakes are present.	- Shampoos such as Zinc pyrethrone or ketoconazole 2% shampoo
Seborrheic Dermatits	- Seborrheic areas such as eyebrows, glabella, nasolabial folds, post auricular region or front of the chest, inter scapular area or pubic area are involved in addition to the scalp. - Greasy looking scale and erythema of the underlying skin noted.	- Please see Chap. 5, "Eczema" for details on management of Seborrheic dermatitis
Psoriasis	- Erythematous plaques with adherent silvery scales. Islands of normal skin are usually noted	- Shampoos such as Tar or ketoconazole 2% shampoo & ultra(Super)-potent steroids such as clobetasol propionate 0.05% suspension. If not better systemic treatment can be considered

Table 8.2 Common conditions causing hair loss: Key diagnostic clinical features and their management

Common skin diseases that cause hair loss	Key clinical features that can aid in diagnosis	Management
AGA	- Men: diagnosis quite obvious clinically - Women: gradual reduction of hair density over a period of time - Hair pull test is positive in frontal region but negative in occipital region	Men: minoxidil 5% topical. If refractory Finasteride 1 mg po q daily Women: minoxidil 5% topical. If peripheral excess androgen symptoms noted, Spironolcatone can be given up to 200 mg po q daily
AA	- Circumscribed patches of bald areas noted. Exclamation type of hairs, and nail changes (pitting or sandpaper nails), can help in the diagnosis	Please see the text for details on its management
TE	- Telogen effluvium is usually associated with a precipitating event - Patients often describe losing lot of hair on a daily basis with routine activities such as combing, shampooing - Hair pull test is positive in all areas	Self-limiting once the triggering factor is eliminated
Trichotillomania	- The distribution of hair loss is quite peculiar, occurring in those areas that are easily accessible for pulling one's own hair	Education & underlying treatment of any psychiatric condition

Bibliography

Alkhalifah A. Topical and intralesional therapies for alopecia areata. Dermatol Ther. 2011;24(3):355–63.

American Academy of Dermatology Association. Alopecia areata: diagnosis and treatment [Internet]. American Academy of Dermatology Association; 2023. Available from: https://www.aad.org/public/diseases/hair-loss/types/alopecia/treatment

Asghar F, Shamim N, Farooque U, Sheikh H, Aqeel R. Telogen effluvium: a review of the literature. Cureus. 2020;12(5).

Devjani S, Ezemma O, Kelley KJ, Stratton E, Senna MM. Androgenetic alopecia: therapy update; 2023.

Eisen DB, Asgari MM, Bennett DD, Connolly SM, Dellavalle RP, Freeman EE, et al. Guidelines of care for the management of actinic keratosis. J Am Acad Dermatol [Internet]. 2021. Available from: https://www.jaad.org/article/S0190-9622(21)00502-8/fulltext

Gordon K, Gordon K, Tosti A. Alopecia: evaluation and treatment. Clin Cosmet Investig Dermatol. 2011;101.

Grant JE, Chamberlain SR. Trichotillomania. Am J Psychiatry. 2016;173(9):868–74.

Grover C, Khurana A. Telogen effluvium. Indian J Dermatol Venereol Leprol. 2013;79(5):591.
Gupta AK, Foley KA. 5% Minoxidil: treatment for female pattern hair loss. PubMed. 2015;19(6):5–7.
Irwig MS. Depressive symptoms and suicidal thoughts among former users of finasteride with persistent sexual side effects. J Clin Psychiatry. 2012;73(09):1220–3.
Meah N, Wall D, York K, Bhoyrul B, Bokhari L, Sigall DA, et al. The Alopecia Areata Consensus of Experts (ACE) study: results of an international expert opinion on treatments for alopecia areata. J Am Acad Dermatol [Internet]. 2020;83(1):123–30. Available from: https://pubmed.ncbi.nlm.nih.gov/32165196/
Olsen EA, Dunlap FE, Funicella T, Koperski JA, Swinehart JM, Tschen EH, et al. A randomized clinical trial of 5% topical minoxidil versus 2% topical minoxidil and placebo in the treatment of androgenetic alopecia in men. J Am Acad Dermatol. 2002;47(3):377–85.
Otberg N, Shapiro J. Alopecia areata. In: Kang S, Amagai M, Bruckner AL, Enk AH, Margolis DJ, McMichael AJ, et al., eds. Fitzpatrick's dermatology, 9th ed. McGraw-Hill Education; 2019.
Otberg N, Shapiro J. Cicatricial alopecias. In: Kang S, Amagai M, Bruckner AL, Enk AH, Margolis DJ, McMichael AJ, et al., eds. Fitzpatrick's dermatology, 9th ed. McGraw-Hill Education; 2019.
Phillips TG, Slomiany WP, Allison R. Hair loss: common causes and treatment. Am Fam Physician. 2017;96(6):371–8 PMID: 28925637.
Recabar S. Trichotillomania | DermNet NZ [Internet]; 2016. Available from: https://dermnetnz.org/topics/trichotillomania
Rossi A, Cantisani C, Scarnò M, Trucchia A, Fortuna MC, Calvieri S. Finasteride, 1 mg daily administration on male androgenetic alopecia in different age groups: 10-year follow-up. Dermatol Ther. 2011;24(4):455–61.
Sterkens A, Lambert J, Bervoets A. Alopecia areata: a review on diagnosis, immunological etiopathogenesis and treatment options. Clin Exp Med. 2021.
Thai KE, Fergin P, Freeman M, Vinciullo C, Francis D, Spelman L, et al. A prospective study of the use of cryosurgery for the treatment of actinic keratoses. Int J Dermatol. 2004;43(9):687–92.
Waldman RA, Grant-Kels JM. Dermatology for the primary care provider. Philadelphia, PA: Elsevier; 2021.
Whiting DA. Cicatricial alopecia: clinico-pathological findings and treatment. Clin Dermatol. 2001;19(2):211–25.

Chapter 9
Face

Abstract This chapter provides an overview of the common dermatological conditions such as acne vulgaris, rosacea, perioral dermatitis, contact dermatitis among many others that can occur on the face. The chapter discusses mainly from their clinical perspective. It provides details about the clinical presentation of these conditions and ways to diagnose them; where appropriate it provides clinical information regarding how to diagnose them clinically. It also discusses their treatment options and the circumstances as to when the patients need to be referred to the dermatologist.

Keywords Acne · Rosacea · Perioral dermatitis · Actinic keratosis (AK) · Contact dermatitis · Seborrheic dermatitis · Atopic dermatitis · Psedofolliculitis barbae · Melasma

9.1 Acne Vulgaris

- Acne vulgaris is a chronic inflammatory skin disorder of the pilosebaceous unit (Eichenfield et al. 2021).

- Comedones are the characteristic lesions. They can be closed (white heads) or open (black heads).
  - Cutibacterium acnes is implicated mainly in the pathogenesis of acne vulgaris (Reynolds et al. 2024).

  - The clinical picture could vary depending upon the stage of acne: there could be only comedones or comedones with inflammatory papules or pustules or cystic acne (Figs. 9.1 and 9.2).

  - Face, V area of the chest, back of the trunk and upper arms can be involved (Fig. 9.3). Lesions need not have to involve all the locations. Examining those areas could aid in the diagnosis and also in management.

D. K. Yellumahanthi, *Manual of Primary Care Dermatology*,
https://doi.org/10.1007/978-3-031-68406-7_9

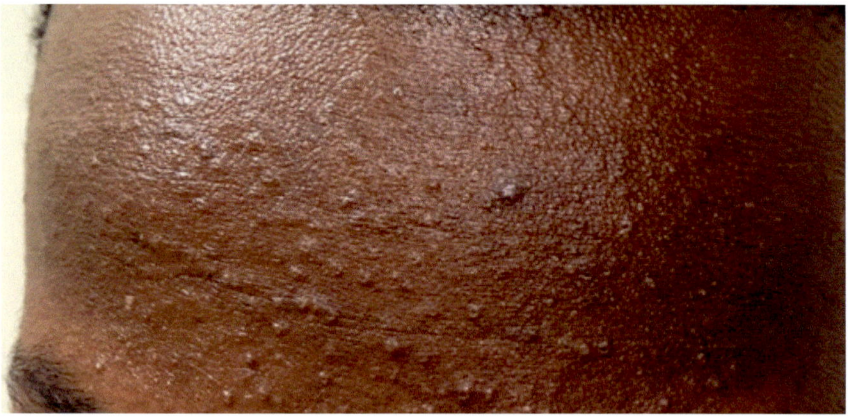

Fig. 9.1 Acne with comedones

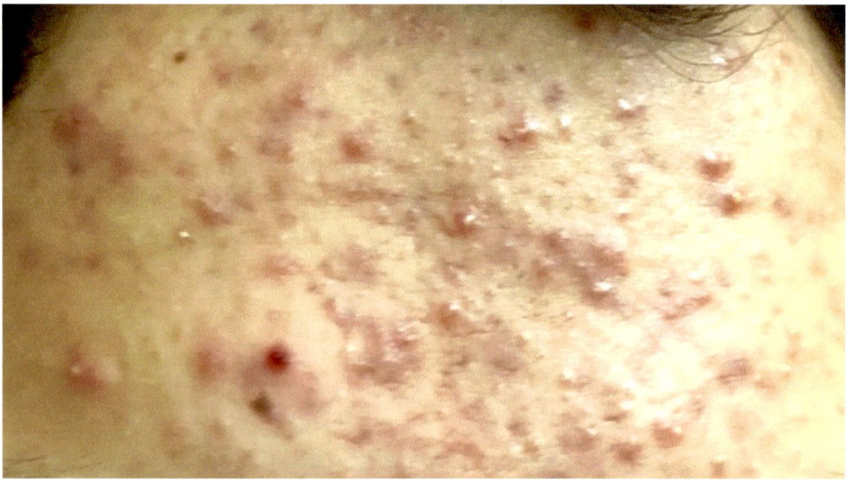

Fig. 9.2 Acne with comedones, papules and pustules

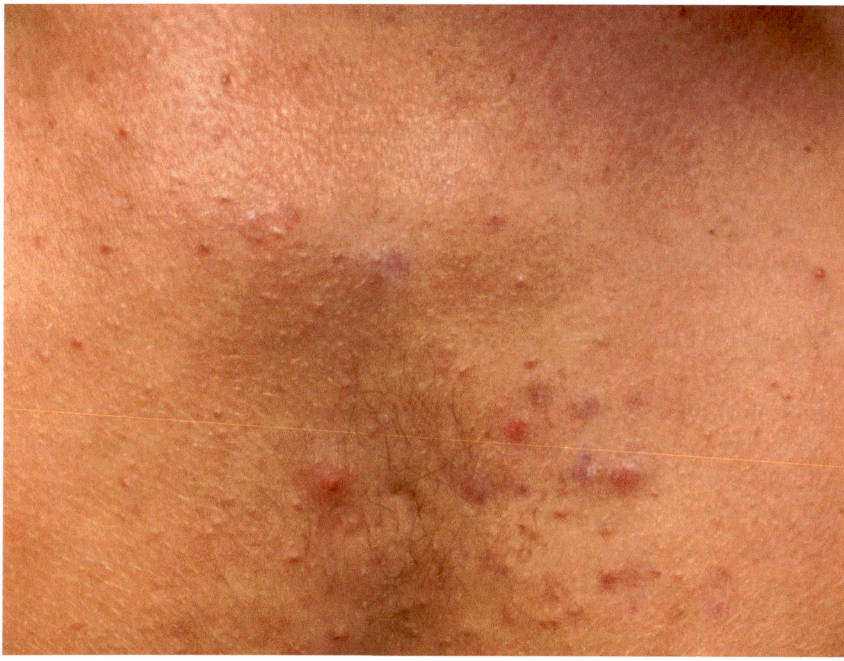

Fig. 9.3 Acne on the chest

9.1.1 *Diagnosis*

- Diagnosis of acne is based on history and physical examination.

9.1.2 *Treatment of Acne*

- Topical therapy, systemic antibiotics, hormonal agents, oral isotretinoin and physical modalities such as comedonal extraction, photodynamic therapy are the various modalities available for the treatment of acne (Reynolds et al. 2024).

Topical Therapy

Among the therapeutics available for acne, topical therapy is the mainstay of acne treatment. common topical agents used include topical retinoids, benzoyl peroxide (BP) and antibiotics.

- **Topical Retinoids**: Topical tretinoin, tazarotene, adapalene and trifarotone are the retinoids that are FDA (Food and Drug Administration) approved for treatment of acne. They are comedolytic and anti-inflammatory and have multiple acne related benefits (Tan et al. 2019). Thus can be used both for comedones and inflammatory lesions.

There is no data currently to suggest superiority of one topical retinoid against another (Reynolds et al. 2024; Shalita et al. 1996).

Retinoids need to be applied in the night time. Patients need to be cautioned regarding avoiding sunlight. Side effects include dryness, exfoliation and burning sensation.

- **Benzoyl Peroxide**: Benzoyl peroxide is mildly comedolytic. It has both inflammatory and non-inflammatory functions (Fulton et al. 1974).

  Side effects include burning sensation, irritation, staining of clothes and bleaching.

- **Topical Antibiotics**: Include clindamycin, erythromycin and minocycline. They are mainly indicated for inflammatory lesions of acne such as papule, pustules (Reynolds et al. 2024).

- **Miscellaneous**: Topical Azelaic acid and topical clascoterone, a topical antiandrogen can also be used (Rosette et al. 2019).

Systemic Antibiotics

- FDA approved antibiotics for acne are doxycycine, minocycline, sarecycline (Reynolds et al. 2024).

- Doxycycline is the commonly used one.

- In view of some potential (rare) side effects of minocycline such as autoimmune hepatitis, skin hyperpigmentation, drug-induced lupus, vertigo and hypersensitivity syndrome. Minocycline is only conditionally recommended to use in acne by the recent American Academy of Dermatology Acne vulgaris guidelines (Reynolds et al. 2024).

- Oral antibiotics are mainly used in moderate to severe acne where predominantly inflammatory lesions are present.

- It is recommended that topical medical therapy is continued while using oral antibiotics. This can help in both decreasing the overall duration of the need for oral antibiotics and also reduce the chances of antibiotic resistance.

- Antibiotics should be limited to no more than 3–4 months at a stretch (Nast et al. 2016; Oon et al. 2019).

Hormonal Agents

- Combined oral contraceptives: In this group the following are FDA approved for treatment of acne in women among those who also desire oral contraception.

  Drospirenone/Ethinyl estradiol.

  Drospirenone/Ethinyl estradiol/levomefolate.

  Norgestimate/Ethinyl estradiol.

  Norethindrone acetate/Ethinyl estradiol/ferrous fumarate (Reynolds et al. 2024).

- Spironolactone:

  It is not FDA approved for the treatment of acne.

  Routine monitoring for potassium may not be needed unless the patient has other risk factors that could predispose for hyperkalemia (Patiyasikunt et al. 2020).

- Intralesional corticosteroid such as triamcinolone has been used as an adjuvant therapy for treating nodules and papules of acne (Reynolds et al. 2024).

Isotretinoin

Scenarios where isotretinoin is used:

- Primarily has been indicated by FDA for use in severe recalcitrant nodular acne (Reynolds et al. 2024).

- Isotretinoin is very effective in the treatment of cystic acne. It reduces the size of sebaceous glands, lowers sebum excretion, regulates cell proliferation and also decreases keratinization (Paichitrojjana and Paichitrojjana 2023).

- It also has been widely used to treat mild to moderate acne that is refractory to other therapies (Agarwal et al. 2011; Akman et al. 2007).
  - The usual dosage of isotretinoin recommended is 0.5 to 1 mg/kg/day in two divided doses.

  - The starting dose is 0.5 mg/kg; and it is increased to 1 mg/kg if patient is tolerating. The duration of therapy is about four to six months with a target cumulative dose of 120–150 mg/kg/course (Dessinioti et al. 2020).

  - Attempt to discontinue the treatment should be considered if the clinical severity score of acne has improved more than 90% compared to the beginning of treatment (Layton 2009).

- **Adverse Effects**: They can be divided broadly into cutaneous and extra cutaneous.

  Among cutaneous side effects, dryness and desquamation of the skin and mucous membranes are common side effects: Cheilitis (90–100% of individuals) is the most common mucocutaneous adverse event (Ornelas et al. 2015).

  If the dose is too high, it can cause dryness of nose and eyes (Villani et al. 2022).

  Extracutaneous: It is teratogenic. A pregnancy test before beginning therapy and monthly thereafter is usually required. Female patient is advised to use a safe contraceptive method during and for 1 month after stopping the therapy.

  Depression is another important side effect.

  Dry eye disease, blepharoconjunctivitis, chalazion are common adverse eye events reported (Villani et al. 2022).

  Low back pain is another common side effect.

- Although there are no published guidelines regarding detailed recommendations on laboratory monitoring during isotretinoin therapy, lipids and hepatic enzymes, at baseline and at month 1 and 3 thereafter must be evaluated when using isotretinoin (Isotretinoin 2019; Cleach et al. 2017; Asai et al. 2015).

- In the USA, registering for pregnancy prevention program iPLEDGE is mandatory (Zaenglein et al. 2016).

- The iPledge program requires women of childbearing potential to abstain or commit to use at least two forms of contraception for the total duration of therapy and also for at least for one month after the end of the isotretinoin treatment (Villani et al. 2022).

- Two negative pregnancy tests 1 month apart before starting isotretinoin, and monthly thereafter is the norm (Landis 2020).

The above is the summary of therapeutics available for acne. Among all these, the recent American Academy of Dermatology (AAD) guidelines for Acne vulgaris have strong recommendations for topical benzoyl peroxide, topical antibiotics, topical retinoids and for oral doxycycline. Oral isotretinoin is also strongly recommended for severe acne and recalcitrant acne after using standard therapy (Reynolds et al. 2024).

9.2 Rosacea

- More common in adults.

- Could manifest initially as episodic flushing and transient erythema. Later may develop persistent erythema, papules, pustules, telengectasia (Figs. 9.4, 9.5 and 9.6). Not all cases have all these lesions. Characteristic nose involvement called rhinophyma can also occur.

- Ocular involvement is common in about 58–72% of the cases. Symptoms of ocular rosacea include foreign body sensation, redness, burning, itching and blurred vision. Blepharitis is common. Both the eyes are usually affected (Vieira and Mannis 2013).

- Facial distribution most often involves the nose, cheeks and chin. Nasolabial folds are spared.

- Episodes may be triggered by spicy foods, hot beverages, alcohol, chocolate, extreme temperatures changes, stress and contact with demodex species (Waldman and Grant-Kels 2022).

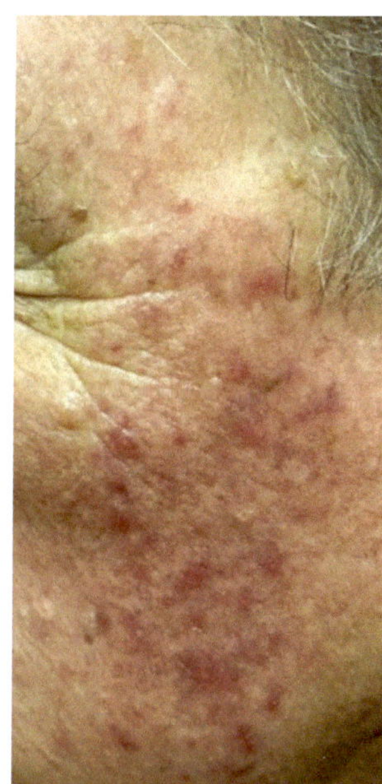

Fig. 9.4 Rosacea with papules

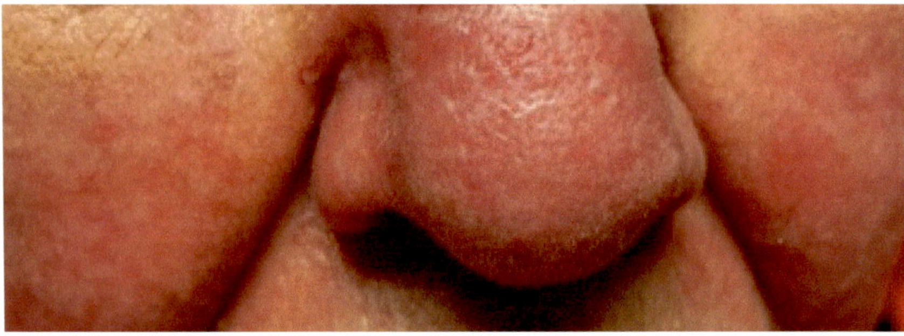

Fig. 9.5 Rosacea with persistent erythema

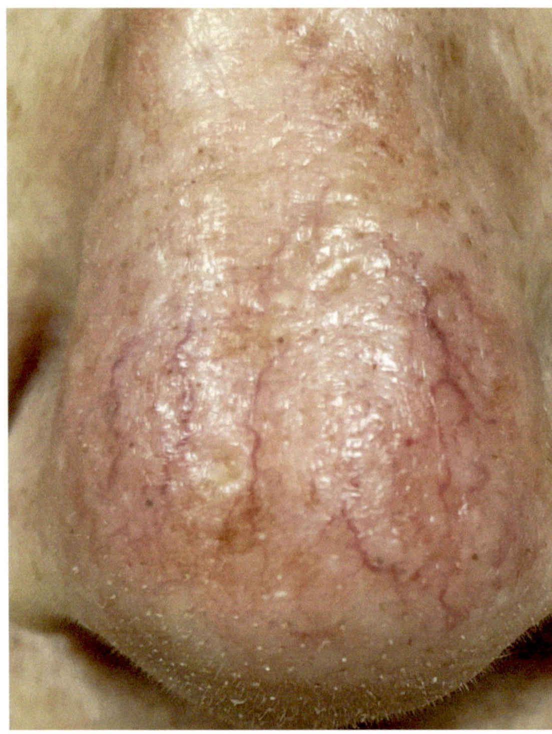

Fig. 9.6 Rosacea with telengectasia

9.2.1 Diagnosis

– Diagnosis is based on clinical history and physical examination. Absence of comedones differentiates from acne. Also, presence of telengectasia (if present) and symptoms such as flushing helps differentiate from acne.

9.2.2 Management

- Avoidance of triggers is very important step.
- Sunscreen with SPF > 30 to be used daily.
- Papulo pustular type has better results with medications.
- In general, for mild papulo pustular lesions topical medications such as ivermectin (1%), metronidazole (0.75%–1%), azelaic acid (15%) can be used. For moderate to severe lesions, combination with oral doxycycline or minocycline can be given.
- If there is only persistent erythema, topical brimonidine 0.33% gel or oxymetazoline 1% cream can be prescribed (van Zuuren 2017).
- Flushing may be treated adults with clonidine 0.05 mg twice daily orally or beta-blockers (Waldman and Grant-Kels 2022). Moderate to severe ocular rosacea can respond to oral tetracyclines (Vieira and Mannis 2013).
- For telengectasia, laser therapy can be tried.
- Rhinophymatous changes can be amenable to surgery or laser.

9.3 Perioral Dermatitis

- Perioral dermatitis is often manifested as erythematous papules or pustule around the oral cavity (Fig. 9.7). Vermilion border tends to be spared (Tolaymat and Hall 2024).
- It can also manifest around the eyes and around the nose.
- Usually asymptomatic.
- It is predominantly common in females. Usually more common between the age group 20–45 years (Lipozencic and Ljubojevic 2011).
- The exact etiology is idiopathic although several are linked to its possible etiology. Among them, the foremost important is usage of topical steroids on the face (Ljubojeviae et al. 2002).

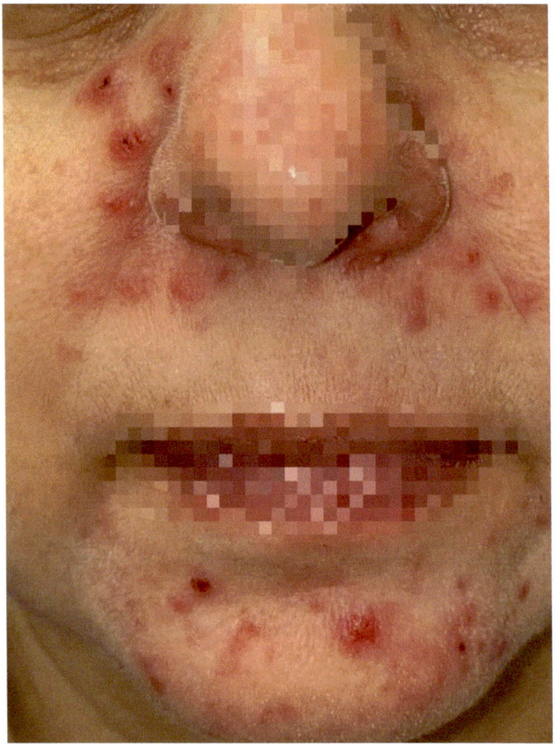

Fig. 9.7 Perioral dermatitis. Note the sparing of vermilion border

- There are also reports of its association with nasal and inhaled corticosteroids (Tolaymat and Hall 2024).

9.3.1 Diagnosis

- Clinical. History and the physical examination can help in making the diagnosis. Rosacea and acne come under differential diagnosis. Absence of comedones excludes acne. Rosacea predominantly involves centro facial area and if symptoms such as flushing are present that points toward the diagnosis of rosacea. It is also important to know that some view perioral dermatitis as a variant of Rosacea.

9.3.2 Management

- Stop the topical steroids if patient happens to be using.

- For mild cases, topical treatment should suffice. Treatment options include erythromycin 2% gel; metronidazole 1% (cream, gel), clindamycin 1% gel and topical azelaic acid (Tolaymat and Hall 2024; Jansen 2004).

- Topical calcineurin inhibitors such as pimecrolimus 1% cream can also be used (Chu 2005).

- Moderate and severe cases may need supplementation with oral antibiotics. Doxycycline 100 mg daily, erythromycin 800 mg daily, clarithromycin 250 mg daily are among the antibiotics used (Searle et al. 2021).

- The disease can be associated with remissions and exacerbations.

9.4 Atopic Dermatitis (AD) (Fig. 9.8)

- AD is more common in children. It could be associated with Allergic rhinitis, asthma.

- It is a chronic pruritic relapsing disorder.

- The clinical appearance of AD depends on age of the patient:
  Mainly facial and extensor involvement in infancy.
  Manifests as flexural eczema (or lichenification) in children and adults.

- AD may subside as the patient grows older. However, they tend to be prone to itching and inflammation when exposed to exogenous irritants.

- In the adults, somtimes AD can manifest as localized dermatitis, like hand dermatitis, nipple, or eyelid eczema.

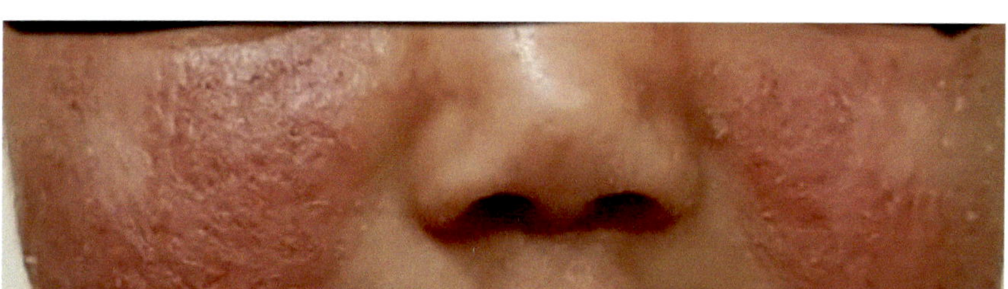

Fig. 9.8 Atopic dermatitis. Courtesy: Dr. P. V. Krishna Rao, Dermatologist, India

- **Management**: Avoidance of triggers and usage of emollients are the cornerstone of the treatment. Topical steroids can be used for the flare ups. Calcineurone inhibitors are a good option for maintenance.

- Please see Chap. 5, 'Eczema' for more details regarding its clinical presentation, diagnosis and management.

9.5 Contact Dermatitis (Fig. 9.9)

- It is quite common on the face.

- The clinical presentation of contact dermatitis varies depending on the likely cause of exposure and the specific body region. For instance, a hairline pattern that affects the superior forehead and nape of the neck could be caused by perming solutions and dyes (Waldman and Grant-Kels 2022).

- Similarly, isolated involvement of both cheeks can be due to the application of any cosmetics to that area.

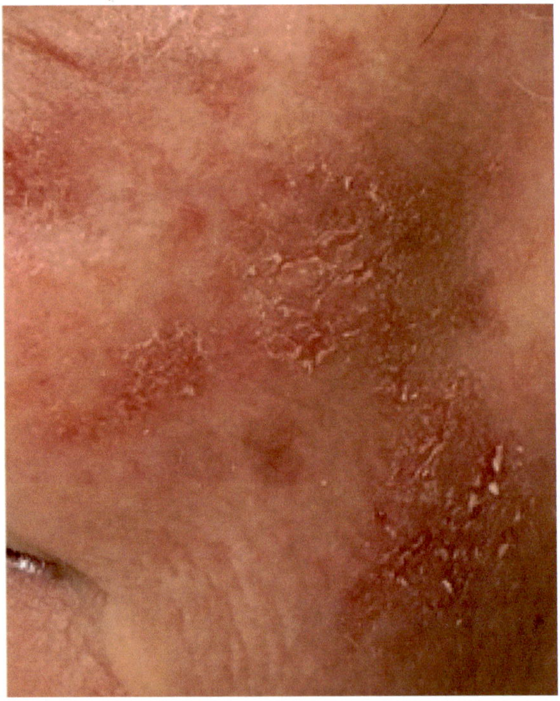

Fig. 9.9 Contact dermatitis on the cheek

- Contact dermatitis to nail polish can manifest as isolated involvement of eyelids. Exposure to airborne allergens can involve the upper eyelids, nasolabial fold and submental area (Waldman and Grant-Kels 2022).

- The usual clinical picture is in the form of erythematous patches with some dryness. Unlike seborrheic dermatitis, does not have to confine itself to seborrheic areas.

9.5.1 Management

- The initial approach of contact dermatitis includes identification of the potential allergen and avoiding it. A detailed history of all the cosmetics that patient has been using on the face including sunscreens need to be sought.

- Any cleansing products, hair products, cosmetics or airborne allergens can cause contact dermatitis on the face (Waldman and Grant-Kels 2022).

- Also, see if the patient is wearing nail polish. Sometimes scratching the face with the nail, can lead to the contact of the nail polish onto the face and can cause allergic dermatitis kind of manifestations on the face.

- Low potent topical steroid like desonide 0.05% cream can be used for few days if needed.

- If the patient is having persistence of symptoms or the rash is recurring, referral to dermatology would be warranted for patch testing and further evaluation.

9.6 Actinic Keratosis

- Actinic keratoses (AK) are the most common epithelial precancerous lesions. They have the potential for malignant transformation to cutaneous squamous cell cancer (SCC). Therefore, treatment or close monitoring is recommended (Waldman and Grant-Kels 2021).

- AK are most commonly seen on chronically sun exposed surfaces of the face, ears, balding scalp, dorsal hands and forearms.

- Commonly, they present as multiple, discrete, flat or elevated, keratotic skin-colored of size measuring between 3 mm to 1 cm in diameter (Fig. 9.10).

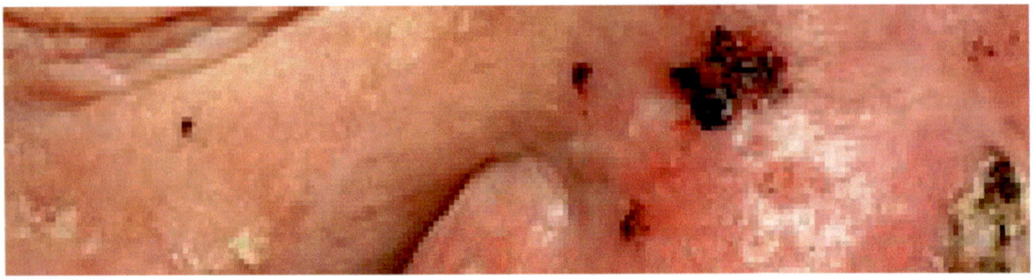

Fig. 9.10 Actinic keratosis lesions are noted on the left side

9.6.1 Management

- The most important step in management is to prevent further sun damage (Waldman and Grant-Kels 2021).

- Cryotherapy with liquid nitrogen is most effective and practical of treating AK when there are a limited number of lesions. A single freeze–thaw cycle of 5 to 10 seconds with open spray technique is often the treatment recommended (Primary Care Dermatology Society).

- Hypertrophic AK may need long duration of freeze times.

- For extensive, broad or numerous lesions, field therapy with either topical chemotherapy or photodynamic therapy (PDT) is recommended.

- 5-FU cream, 0.5–5%, or imiquimod 5% cream are the two chemotherapeutic agents used for field therapy. Other agents approved are diclofenac 3% gel & tirbanibulin.

- Please see Chap. 8, 'Scalp' for more details on clinical features and management of AK.

9.7 Phtosensitivity Rash

- It normally manifests as erythematous patches or papules more so in the malar region of the face. However, any part of the face can be involved.

- Typical history is that the rash gets worse when going outdoors and exposed to the sunlight. Sometimes also complains of having burning sensation or itching when goes in to the sun.

- When photosensitivity rash is suspected, systemic conditions that can cause photosensitivity need to be ruled out. For example, connective tissue disorders like lupus. Also, make sure patient is not taking any drugs that can cause photosensitivity. For example doxycycline.

- If no systemic conditions are identified, the management is done empirically. Strict avoidance of sunlight or using of sunscreen is vital for management. Mild potent topical steroids like desonide 0.05% cream can be used for few days if needed.

9.8 Cutaneous Infections

- Angular cheilitis (Fig. 9.11)

- Could be due to candida if the angle of the lips is moist and red. KOH preparation reveals candida pseudohyphae.

- **Treatment**: Topical nystatin or clotrimazole. Systemic therapy with oral fluconazole if needed.

- Besides angular cheilitis, many other infections such as herpes simplex labialis, tinea facei or barbae, Shingles, Warts, cellulitis, folliculitis, furuncle, abscess can occur on the face. Please see Chap. 6, 'Common Cutaneous Infections' for etiology, clinical presentation, diagnosis and management of these conditions.

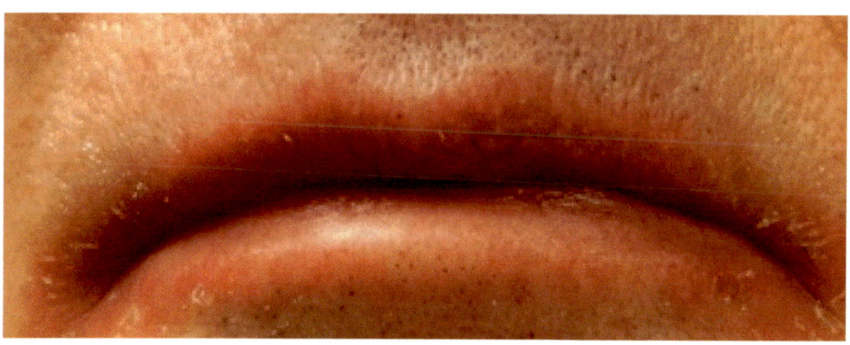

Fig. 9.11 Angular cheilitis

9.9 Pseudofolliculitis Barbae

- Pseudofolliculitis barbae is a chronic inflammatory disorder manifested with papules that are caused due to ingrowing of the curved shaft of the hair.

- Secondary infection can cause pustules as well.

- More common in African American and Asian Americans (Ogunbiyi 2019).

- It usually occurs in the lower beard area (Ogunbiyi 2019).

9.9.1 Management

- Acute inflammation: Temporary cessation of shaving helps and is recommended (Primary Care Dermatology Society) along with other palliative measures.

- For moderate to severe inflammatory lesions, topical corticosteroids, antibiotics and benzyl peroxide has been found useful either as monotherapy or in combination (Bridgeman-Shah 2004; Cook-Bolden et al. 2004). Intralesional corticosteroids can also be used for short periods to reduce inflammation.

- Topical retinoids and glycolic acid preparations have also been useful (Kligman and Mills 1973; Coley and Alexis 2009).

- Prevention: Although cessation of shaving helps it may not be practically feasible.

  Shaving with electric clippers with gauge set such that at least 1mm of the hair is left behind, helps (Alexander 1981; Al et al. 1978).

9.10 Seborrheic Dermatitis

- Please see Chap. 5, 'Eczema' for more details regarding its clinical presentation, diagnosis and management.

9.11 Discoid Lupus Erythematosus (DLE) (Fig. 9.12)

- Please see Chap. 3, 'Papulosquamous Disorders' for more details regarding the clinical presentation, diagnosis and management of DLE.

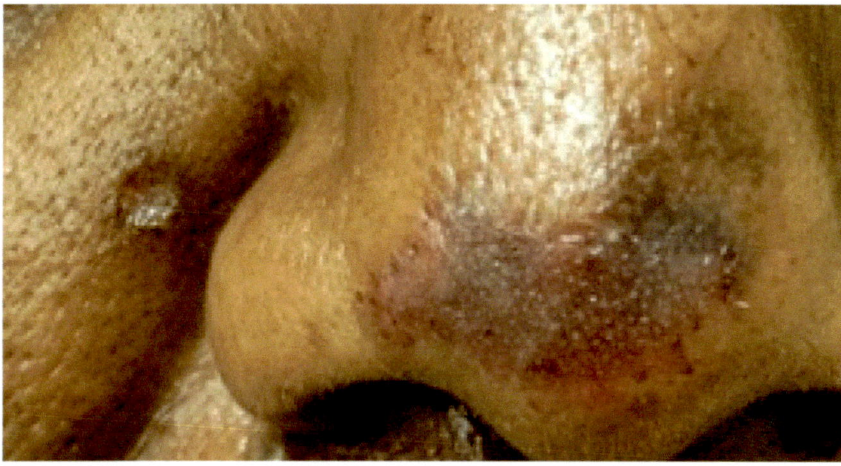

Fig. 9.12 Discoid lupus erythematosus

9.12 Melasma (Fig. 9.13)

- Melasma is manifested by asymmetric, irregular, brown-colored, macules/patches on either face (most common) or other sun exposed areas of the skin (Kwon et al. 2019).

Fig. 9.13 Melasma on the cheek

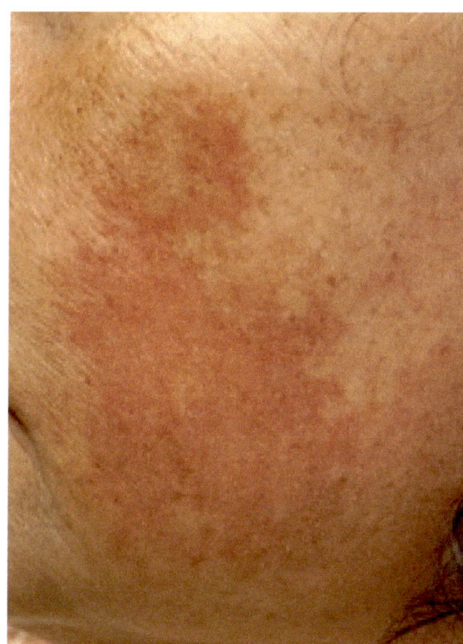

- It is an acquired pigmentary disorder (Passeron and Picardo 2018).

- It gets worse during summer months (Passeron and Picardo 2018). It is due to female hormone stimulation in a genetically predisposed individual and UV light is a triggering factor (Passeron and Picardo 2018).

9.12.1 Management

- Treatment is challenging. There is no single effective treatment available. Among the medical treatments, triple combination of hydroquinone, corticosteroid and retinoic acid (Kligman formula) is the most effective treatment (Chan et al. 2008).

- Sunprotection needs to be recommended. Sunscreens that block shorter wavelength in addition to UVA and UVB is found to be more protective than only those that are just broad spectrum (Boukari et al. 2015).

- Cases not responding to the above measures, can be referred to a dermatologist for trying other therapeutic options.

Bibliography

Agarwal US, Besarwal RK, Bhola K. Oral isotretinoin in different dose regimens for acne vulgaris: a randomized comparative trial. Indian J Dermatol Venereol Leprol [Internet]. 2011;77(6):688–94. Available from: https://www.ncbi.nlm.nih.gov/pubmed/22016276

Akman A, Durusoy C, Senturk M, Koc CK, Soyturk D, Alpsoy E. Treatment of acne with intermittent and conventional isotretinoin: a randomized, controlled multicenter study. Arch Dermatol Res [Internet]. 2007;299(10):467–73. Available from: https://pubmed.ncbi.nlm.nih.gov/17710426/

Al H, Garcia RL, Garcia RL, Henderson AL. The adjustable rotary electric razor in the control of Pseudofolliculitis barbae. J Assoc Mil Dermatol. 1978;4:28.

Alexander AM. Evaluation of a foil-guarded shaver in the management of pseudofolliculitis barbae. Cutis. 1981;27(5):534–42.

Asai Y, Baibergenova A, Dutil M, Humphrey S, Hull P, Lynde C, et al. Management of acne: Canadian clinical practice guideline. Can Med Assoc J [Internet]. 2015;188(2):118–26. Available from: http://www.cmaj.ca/content/188/2/118 [cited 2019 Feb 28].

Boukari F, Jourdan E, Fontas E, Montaudié H, Castela E, Lacour JP, et al. Prevention of melasma relapses with sunscreen combining protection against UV and short wavelengths of visible light: a prospective randomized comparative trial. J Am Acad Dermatol [Internet]. 2015;72(1):189–90.e1. Available from: https://pubmed.ncbi.nlm.nih.gov/25443629/

Bridgeman-Shah S. The medical and surgical therapy of pseudofolliculitis barbae. Dermatol Ther. 2004;17(2):158–63.

Chan R, Park KC, Lee MH, Lee E-S, Chang SE, Leow YH, et al. A randomized controlled trial of the efficacy and safety of a fixed triple combination (fluocinolone acetonide 001, hydroquinone 4, tretinoin 005) compared with hydroquinone 4 cream in Asian patients with moderate to severe melasma. Br J Dermatol. 2008;159(3):697–703.

Chu C-Y. The use of 1% pimecrolimus cream for the treatment of steroid-induced rosacea. Br J Dermatol. 2005;152(2):396–9.

Le Cleach L, Lebrun-Vignes B, Bachelot A, Beer F, Berger P, Brugère S, et al. Guidelines for the management of acne: recommendations from a French multidisciplinary group. Br J Dermatol [Internet]. 2017;177(4):908–13. Available from: https://academic.oup.com/bjd/article/177/4/908/6674084?login=false [cited 2023 Feb 18].

Coley MK, Alexis AF. Managing common dermatoses in skin of color. Semin Cutan Med Surg. 2009;28(2):63–70.

Cook-Bolden FE, Barba A, Halder R, Taylor S. Twice-daily applications of benzoyl peroxide 5% clindamycin 1%gel versus vehicle in the treatment of pseudofolliculitis barbae. Cutis. 2004;73(Suppl):18–24.

Cryosurgery (also known as cryotherapy) [Internet]. Primary Care Dermatology Society. Available from: https://www.pcds.org.uk/clinical-guidance/cryosurgery-2

Dessinioti C, Zouboulis CC, Bettoli V, Rigopoulos D. Comparison of guidelines and consensus articles on the management of patients with acne with oral isotretinoin. J Eur Acad Dermatol Venereol. 2020;34(10):2229–40.

Eichenfield DZ, Sprague J, Eichenfield LF. Management of acne vulgaris: a review. JAMA [Internet]. 2021;326(20):2055–67. Available from: https://jamanetwork.com/journals/jama/article-abstract/2786495 [cited 2022 Apr 13].

Fulton JE, Farzad-Bakshandeh A, Bradley S. Studies on the mechanism of action of topical benzoyl peroxide and vitamin A acid in acne vulgaris. J Cutan Pathol. 1974;1(5):191–200.

Isotretinoin. Annex I, II, III. European Medicines Agency (EMEA); 2019. Available from: https://www.ema.europa.eu/en/documents/referral/roaccutane-article-30-referral-annex-i-ii-iii_en.pdf [cited 2019 May 19].

Jansen T. Azelaic acid as a new treatment for perioral dermatitis: results from an open study. Br J Dermatol Suppl. 2004;151(4):933–4.

Kligman AM, Mills OH Jr. Pseudofolliculitis of the beard and topically applied tretinoin. Arch Dermatol. 1973;107(4):551–2.

Kwon S-H, et al. Melasma: updates and perspectives. Exp Dermatol. 2019;28(6):704–8. https://doi.org/10.1111/exd.13844.

Landis MN. Optimizing isotretinoin treatment of acne: update on current recommendations for monitoring, dosing, safety, adverse effects, compliance, and outcomes. Am J Clin Dermatol. 2020.

Layton A. The use of isotretinoin in acne. Dermato-Endocrinology [Internet]. 2009;1(3):162–9. Available from: https://www.ncbi.nlm.nih.gov/pmc/articles/PMC2835909/

Lipozencic J, Ljubojevic S. Perioral dermatitis. Clin Dermatol [Internet]. 2011;29(2):157–61. Available from: https://www.sciencedirect.com/science/article/abs/pii/S0738081X10001598

Ljubojeviae S, Basta-Juzbasiae A, Lipozenèiae J. Steroid dermatitis resembling rosacea: aetiopathogenesis and treatment. J Eur Acad Dermatol Venereol. 2002,16(2):121 6.

Nast A, Dréno B, Bettoli V, Bukvic Mokos Z, Degitz K, Dressler C, et al. European evidence-based (S3) guideline for the treatment of acne—update 2016—short version. J Eur Acad Dermatol Venereol. 2016;30(8):1261–8.

Ogunbiyi A. Pseudofolliculitis barbae; current treatment options. Clin Cosmet Investig Dermatol [Internet]. 2019;12:241–7. Available from: https://www.ncbi.nlm.nih.gov/pmc/articles/PMC6585396/

Oon HH, Wong SN, Aw DCW, Cheong WK, Goh CL, Tan HH. Acne management guidelines by the Dermatological Society of Singapore. J Clin Aesthet Dermatol. 2019;12(7):34–50. Epub 2019 Jul 1. PMID: 31531161; PMCID: PMC6715335.

Ornelas J, Rosamilia L, Larsen L, Foolad N, Wang Q, Li CS, et al. Objective assessment of isotretinoin-associated cheilitis: Isotretinoin Cheilitis Grading Scale. J Dermatol Treat. 2015;27(2):153–5.

Paichitrojjana A, Paichitrojjana A. Oral isotretinoin and its uses in dermatology: a review. Drug Des Dev Ther. 2023;17:2573–91.

Passeron T, Picardo M. Melasma, a photoaging disorder. Pigment Cell Melanoma Res. 2018;31(4):461–5.

Patiyasikunt M, Chancheewa B, Asawanonda P, Noppakun N, Kumtornrut C. Efficacy and tolerability of low-dose spironolactone and topical benzoyl peroxide in adult female acne: a randomized, double-blind, placebo-controlled trial. J Dermatol. 2020;47(12):1411–6.

Reynolds RV, Yeung H, Cheng CE, Cook-Bolden F, Desai SR, Druby K, et al. Guidelines of care for the management of acne vulgaris. J Am Acad Dermatol. 2024.

Rosette C, Agan FJ, Mazzetti A, Moro L, Gerloni M. Cortexolone 17α-propionate (clascoterone) is a novel androgen receptor antagonist that inhibits production of lipids and inflammatory cytokines from sebocytes in vitro. J Drugs Dermatol. 2019;18(5):412–8 PMID: 31141847.

Searle T, Ali FR, Al-Niaimi F. Perioral dermatitis: diagnosis, proposed etiologies, and management. J Cosmet Dermatol. 2021.

Shalita A, Weiss JS, Chalker DK, Ellis CN, Greenspan A, Katz HI, et al. A comparison of the efficacy and safety of adapalene gel 0.1% and tretinoin gel 0.025% in the treatment of acne vulgaris: a multicenter trial. J Am Acad Dermatol [Internet]. 1996;34(3):482–5. Available from: https://www.ncbi.nlm.nih.gov/pubmed/8609263

Tan J, Thiboutot D, Popp G, Gooderham M, Lynde C, Rosso JD, et al. Randomized phase 3 evaluation of trifarotene 50 μg/g cream treatment of moderate facial and truncal acne. J Am Acad Dermatol [Internet]. 2019;80(6):1691–9. Available from: https://www.jaad.org/article/S0190-9622(19)30335-4/fulltext [cited 2020 Jun 12].

Tolaymat L, Hall MR. Perioral dermatitis. In: StatPearls [Internet]. Treasure Island (FL): StatPearls Publishing; 2024. PMID: 30247843.

van Zuuren EJ. Rosacea. In: Solomon CG, editor. N Engl J Med 2017;377(18):1754–64.

Vieira AC, Mannis MJ. Ocular rosacea: common and commonly missed. J Am Acad Dermatol. 2013;69(6):S36-41.

Villani A, Nastro FF, di Vico F, Fabbrocini G, Annunziata MC, Genco LV. Oral isotretinoin for acne: a complete overview. Expert Opin Drug Saf. 2022;21(8):1027–37.

Waldman RA, Grant-Kels JM. Dermatology for the primary care provider. Elsevier, Inc; 2021.

Waldman RA, Grant-Kels JM. Dermatology for the primary care provider. Philadelphia, PA: Elsevier; 2022.

Zaenglein AL, Pathy AL, Schlosser BJ, Alikhan A, Baldwin HE, Berson DS, et al. Guidelines of care for the management of acne vulgaris. J Am Acad Dermatol [Internet]. 2016;74(5):945–73.e33. Available from: https://www.jaad.org/article/S0190-9622(15)02614-6/fulltext

Chapter 10
Trunk

Abstract Most of the conditions that involve the trunk also involve other parts of the body. This chapter provides a list of the common dermatological conditions such as pityriasis rosea, pityriasis versicolor and contact dermatitis that can involve the trunk and a brief clinically relevant overview of them.

Keywords Acne · Psoriasis · Pityriasis rosea · Pityriasis versicolor · Seborrheic dermatitis · Contact dermatitis · Subacute cutaneous lupus

The following conditions can involve the trunk either in isolation or as a part of manifestation elsewhere on the body. These conditions need to be considered in the differential diagnosis of all skin rashes seen on the trunk.

- Acne.
- Psoriasis.
- Pityriasis rosea.
- Pityriasis versicolor.
- Seborrheic dermatitis.
- Contact dermatitis.
- Cutaneous infections.
- Subacute cutaneous lupus.

D. K. Yellumahanthi, *Manual of Primary Care Dermatology*,
https://doi.org/10.1007/978-3-031-68406-7_10

10.1 Acne Vulgaris

- It is an inflammation of pilosebaceous units.
- Increased sebum production induced by androgens, inflammation, changes in keratinization and colonization of hair follicles by propionobacterium acnes are the main factors that cause it (Williams et al. 2012).
- Propionobacterium is currently called as cutibacterium acnes.
- Common age group—adolescents.
- Although face is the most common area where patients complain of having acne, it can also occur on the back of the trunk and 'V' area of the chest (Figs. 10.1 and 10.2).
- Therefore, in all rashes that occur in these areas, acne needs to be ruled out.
- Comedones, papules, pustules are the common lesions noted in these areas, although nodules and cysts can also occur.
- Please see Chap. 9, 'Face', for more details regarding its clinical presentation, diagnosis and management.

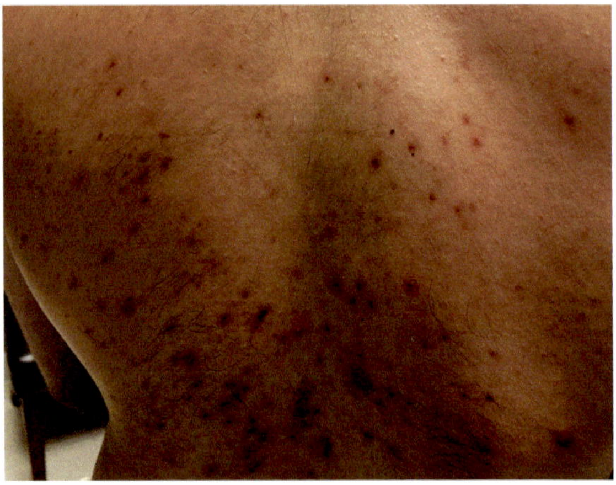

Fig. 10.1 Acne vulgaris involving the back of the trunk

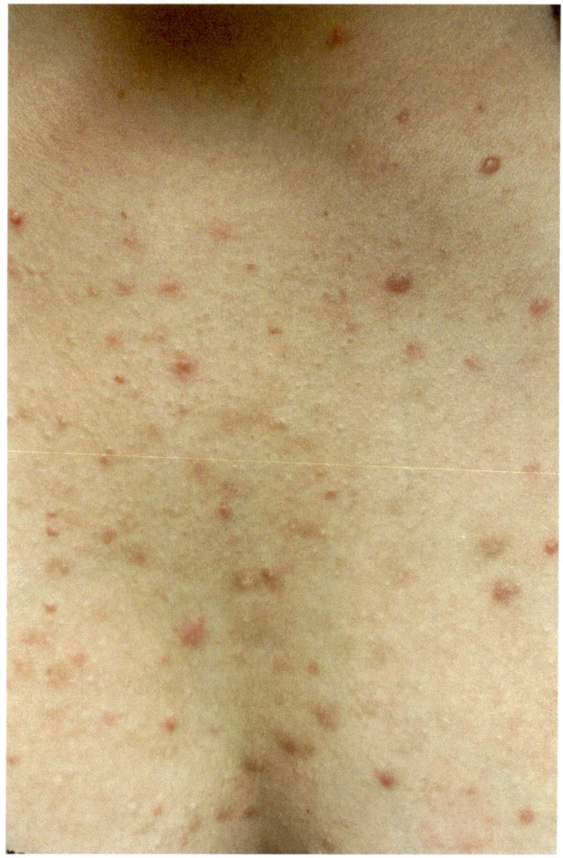

Fig. 10.2 Acne vulgaris involving 'V' area of the chest

10.2 Psoriasis

- Psoriasis is a chronic inflammatory skin disease. It can manifest in a variety of clinical forms. Chronic plaque psoriasis is the most common type of psoriasis. Guttate psoriasis, that manifests as acute onset of several, small, scaly papules and plaques, is another subtype. Guttate psoriasis is preceded by approximately in two third of the cases by pharyngitis or tonsillitis (Griffiths et al. 2021).

- Chronic plaque type usually manifests as erythematous plaques with adherent silvery scales (Fig. 10.3). Common areas of involvement for chronic plaque type are scalp, extensor aspects such as back of the elbow, front of the knee, front of the legs and sacral area. Palms and soles can also be involved. Nail changes such as pitting, transverse and longitudinal ridges can also be noted.

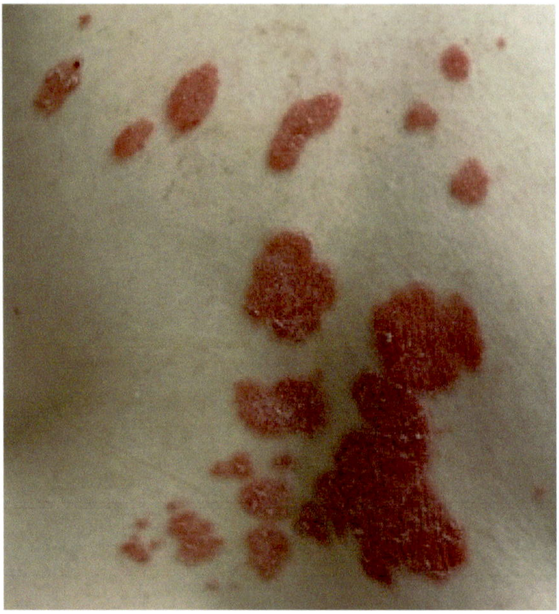

Fig. 10.3 Psoriasis vulgaris on the back of the trunk

- When one area is involved, all the other common areas also need to be examined. Although all the common areas need not have to be involved, presence of similar lesions in more than one of these common areas can increase the suspicion of the diagnosis of psoriasis.

- Please see Chap. 3, 'Papulosquamous disorders', for more details about clinical presentation, diagnosis and management of psoriasis.

10.3 Pityriasis Rosea (PR)

- Please see Chap. 3, 'Papulosquamous disorders", for clinical presentation, diagnosis and management of pityriasis rosea.

10.4 Pityriasis Versicolor (Figs. 10.4 and 10.5)

- Pityriasis versicolor, also known as tinea versicolor, is a superficial fungal infection caused by Malassezia species, which is a yeast that colonizes naturally on the skin surface (Gupta and Lyons 2014).

- Please see Chap. 3, 'Papulosquamous disorders', for details about clinical presentation, diagnosis and management of Pityriasis versicolor.

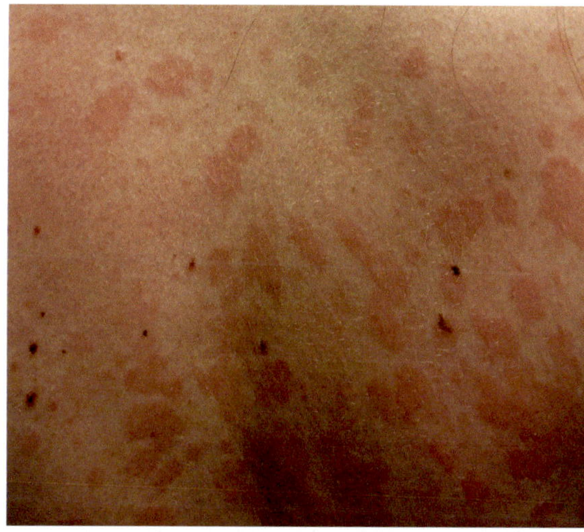

Fig. 10.4 Pityriasis versicolor, manifesting as pink patches

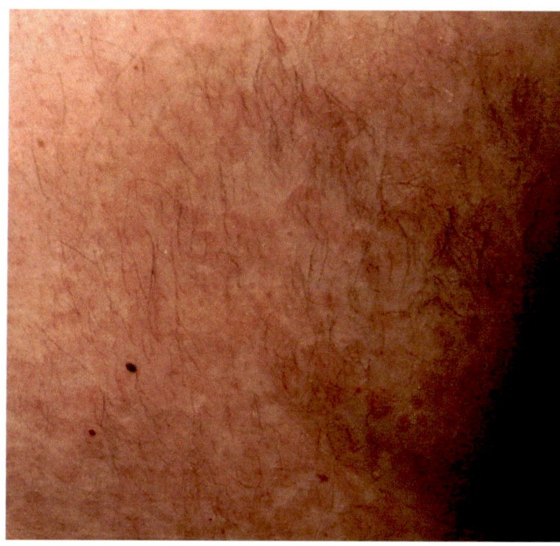

Fig. 10.5 Pityriasis versicolor, manifesting as hyperpigmented patches

10.5 Cutaneous Infections

– Besides, pityriasis versicolor, any infections described in Chap. 6 'Common Cutaneous Infections', can occur on the trunk. More so, scabies and extensive tinea corporis definitely needs to be ruled out, in any extensive skin eruption on the trunk.

10.5.1 *Tinea Corporis*

- Superficial fungal infection of the body.
- Caused by dermatophytes (Yee and Al Aboud 2023).
- The lesions of tinea corporis have raised border with central clearing. Fine scaling is also present (Figs. 10.6 and 10.7).
- Please make sure that the complete cutaneous examination is done to see if similar lesions are present elsewhere with special attention to those areas where tinea corporis is common—axilla, inframammary area in females, groins, nails and feet.
- **Treatment:** Topical antifungals along with oral antifungals when appropriate.
- For the rashes in the inframammary areas, candidiasis, erythrasma and tinea intertrigo need to be ruled out.

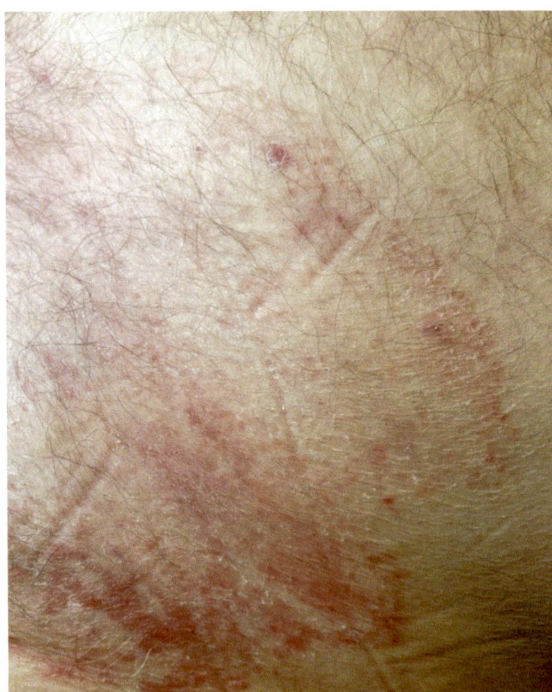

Fig. 10.6 Tinea corporis on the front of the abdomen

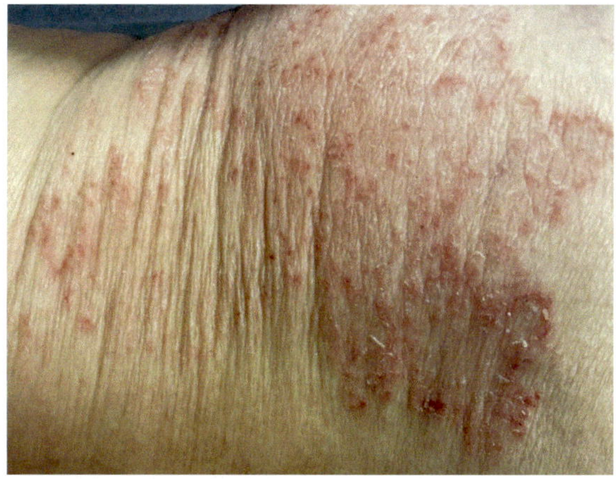

Fig. 10.7 Tinea corporis on the back of the trunk

- Please see Chap. 6 on 'Common Cutaneous Infections' for details on clinical presentation, diagnosis and management of tinea corporis, scabies and other infections mentioned above.

10.6 Seborrheic Dermatitis (SD)

- The exact etiology is multifactorial.

- Malasseizia, the normal body yeast is the likely the cause of seborrheic dermatitis.

- SD is considered as an inflammatory response to Malassezia species (Borda et al. 2019).

- It manifests as erythematous plaques with greasy-looking scales that involves the seborrheic areas such as front of the chest (Fig. 10.8).

- Not always all the seborrheic areas are involved. However, examination of all the seborrheic areas needs to be done anytime seborrheic dermatitis is suspected on the trunk.

- Please see Chap. 5, 'Eczema' for more details on its clinical presentation, diagnosis and management.

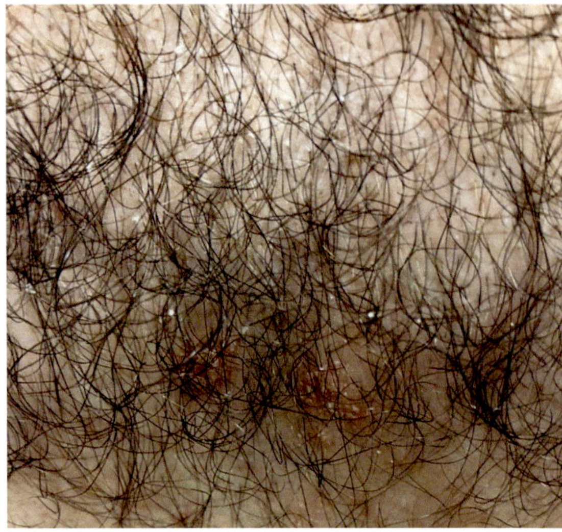

Fig. 10.8 Seborrheic dermatitis

10.7 Contact Dermatitis

- Nickel allergy and allergy to textile products are among others that can cause contact dermatitis on the trunk.

- Nickel allergy is very common. Among many others, nickel is an ingredient in the jean buttons and bra hooks. Therefore, any rashes that are in the vicinity of bra hooks and jean buttons (Fig. 10.9) need to be ruled out for nickel allergy.

- Please see Chap. 5, 'Eczema', for more details on clinical presentation, diagnosis and management of contact dermatitis.

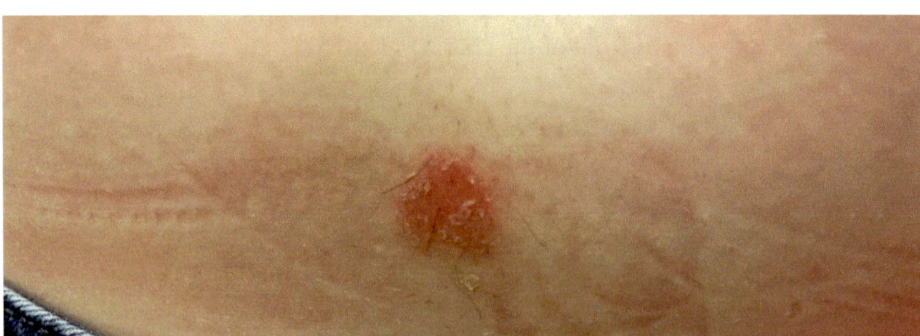

Fig. 10.9 Contact dermatitis to jean button. Likely due to nickel allergy

10.8 Subacute Cutaneous Lupus Erythematosus (SCLE)

- The eruption appears in a photodistributed fashion. Scaly lesions or annular or polycyclic lesions appear in the sun-exposed areas such as V of the chest and upper back (Figs. 10.10 and 10.11). Similar lesions can also be seen on extensor aspects of upper extremities.

- **Management**: Management includes photoprotection, topical potent corticosteroids, topical calcineurin inhibitors and/or systemic glucocorticoids depending on the extent of involvement and subset of disease. Recommend patients of SCLE can be referred to either a dermatologist and/or rheumatologist to rule out systemic

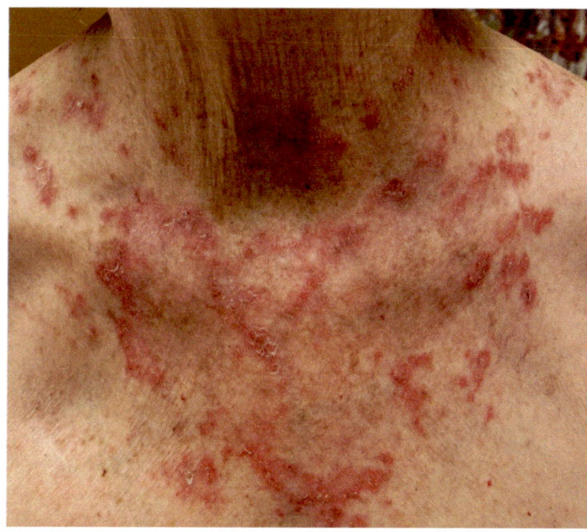

Fig. 10.10 Subacute cutaneous lupus erythematosus involving V area of the chest

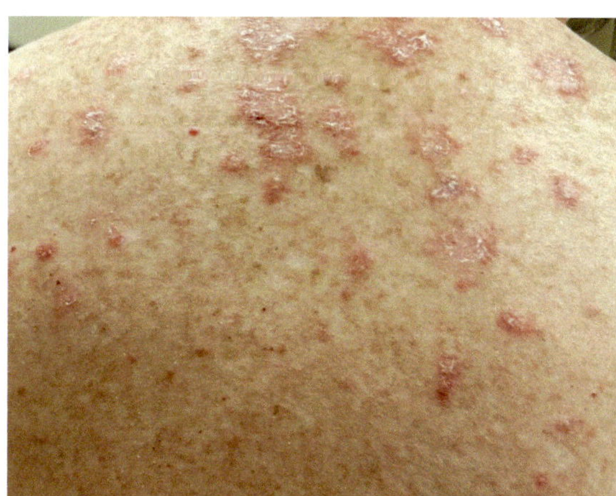

Fig. 10.11 Subacute cutaneous lupus erythematosus involving the upper back of the trunk that is usually exposed to sun

lupus erythematosus (SLE) and the need for hydroxychloroquine for long time management.

– Please see Chap. 3, 'Papulosquamous Disorders', for more details on clinical presentation, diagnosis and management of SCLE.

Bibliography

Borda LJ, Perper M, Keri JE. Treatment of seborrheic dermatitis: a comprehensive review. J Dermatol Treatment. 2019;30(2):158–69. https://www.ncbi.nlm.nih.gov/pubmed/29737895

Griffiths CEM, Armstrong AW, Gudjonsson JE, Barker JNWN. Psoriasis. Lancet. 2021;397(10281):1301–15.

.Gupta AK, Lyons DC. Pityriasis versicolor: an update on pharmacological treatment options. Exp Opin Pharmacother. 2014;15(12):1707–13. https://pubmed.ncbi.nlm.nih.gov/24991691-pityriasis-versicolor-an-update-on-pharmacological-treatment-options/?from_term=%234+AND+%233&from_sort=&from_pos=4&from_exact_term=%28malassezia+furfur%29+AND+%28Pityriasis+versicolor%29

Williams HC, Dellavalle RP, Garner S. Acne vulgaris. Lancet 2012;379(9813):361–72. https://www.sciencedirect.com/science/article/pii/S0140673611603218

Yee G, Al Aboud AM. Tinea corporis. In: StatPearls. Treasure Island (FL). StatPearls Publishing; 2024. https://www.ncbi.nlm.nih.gov/books/NBK544360/

Chapter 11
Upper Extremity Including Hands

Abstract This chapter provides an overview of the common dermatological conditions such as keratosis pilaris, actinic purpura, Actinic keratosis, Granuloma annulare that can involve the upper extremity. The chapter discusses mainly from their clinical perspective. It provides details about the clinical presentation of these conditions and ways to diagnose them; where appropriate it provides clinical information regarding how to diagnose them clinically. It also discusses their treatment options and where appropriate the circumstances as to when the patients need to be referred to the dermatologist.

Keywords Keratosis pilaris · Senile purpura · Actinic keratosis · Atopic dermatitis · Nummular eczema · Psoriasis · Lichen planus · Granuloma annulare · Palmoplantar psoriasis · Pompholyx/dyshyrotic eczema · Hand eczema

Upper Extremity

- Keratosis pilaris.
- Acne.
- Senile purpura.
- Actinic keratosis.
- Eczema.
  - Atopic dermatitis.
  - Nummular eczema
- Psoriasis.
- Lichen planus.
- Cutaneous infections.

D. K. Yellumahanthi, *Manual of Primary Care Dermatology*,
https://doi.org/10.1007/978-3-031-68406-7_11

11.1 Keratosis Pilaris (KP)

- KP is a common and chronic skin disorder that manifests as keratotic follicular papules (Fig. 11.1).
- There could be perifollicular erythema.
- It is common in children.
- Commonly affects the extensor surfaces of arms, buttocks and upper legs (Hosking et al. 2018).
- It's exact etiology is unknown (Hosking et al. 2018).

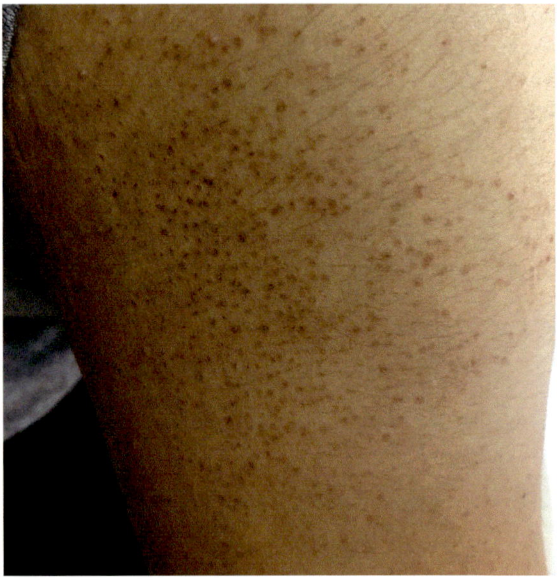

Fig. 11.1 Keratosis pilaris

11.1.1 Diagnosis

- Diagnosis is usually obvious based on clinical examination.

11.1.2 Management

- It has a tendency to improve over the years (Pennycook and McCready 2023). Patients or parents should be made aware of it.

- Emolients and keratolytic preparations containing urea, lactic acid or salicyclic acid can help soften the lesions (Cohen et al. 2020).

- Topical retinoids such as 0.01% tazarotene can also be tried (Gerbig 2002).

- Topical low potent steroids for a brief time can help in relieving the symptoms of itch but do not help in improving the lesions (Bruckner 2019).

11.2 Actinic Purpura or Senile Purpura (Bateman Purpura)

- Acinic purpura commonly manifests in elderly as purpura on the sun exposed areas of the body such as extensor aspects of forearm (Fig. 11.2).

- It is as a result of chronic sun exposure and age related skin thinning. Both these factors make the cutaneous microvasculature fragile to the extent that even minor trauma can lead to extravasation of the blood (Fenske and Lober 1986).

- Drugs such as aspirin and other blood thinners can exacerbate senile purpura (Kerns et al. 2019a).

- Purpura is usually resolved within about 2–3 weeks and often postinflammatory hyperpigmentation may result (Cho et al. 2019b).

Fig. 11.2 Actinic purpura

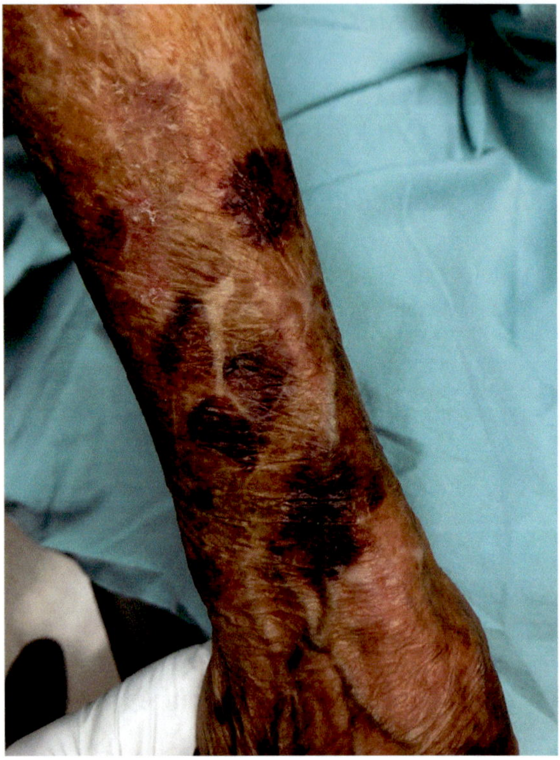

11.2.1 Diagnosis

- In typical cases diagnosis is obvious from history and physical examination. Complete blood count may be done if patient is seen with initial episode to make sure there is no thrombocytopenia. If patient gives history of recurrent episodes that are suggestive of repeated episodes of actinic purpura, then no lab testing is needed.

11.2.2 Management

- Assurance and education about the benign nature of the condition is often adequate.

11.3 Actinic Keratoses (AK)

- Actinic keratoses are neoplasms of keratinocyte occurring on skin that has been chronically exposed to ultraviolet radiation such as face, ears, balding scalp, dorsal hands and forearms (Eisen et al. 2021; Marks et al. 1986; Leonard 2010; Salasche 2000).

- Classically manifests as a rough scaly papule on an erythematous base (Fig. 11.3).

- There are clinical variants such as hypertrophic, atrophic and pigmented. Some of them can develop cutaneous horns.

- The lesions usually measure between 3 mm to 1 cm in diameter, most being less than 6 mm.

- AKs can regress on their own or, can evolve into keratinocyte carcinoma if left untreated (Marks et al. 1988, Elmets et al. 2010; Berman and Cockerell 2013; Czarnecki et al. 2002; Glogau 2000; Mittelbronn et al. 1998).

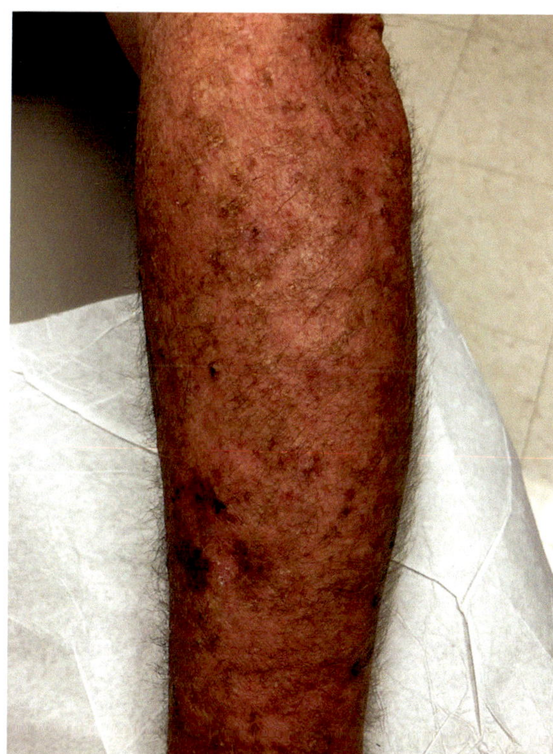

Fig. 11.3 Actinic keratosis

- The estimated risk of progression of AK to SCC vary from less than 0.1% to 20% (Marks et al. 1988; Criscione et al. 2009; Werner et al. 2013).

- Please see Chap. 8, 'Scalp' for more details on clinical presentation, diagnosis and management of AK.

11.4 Acne Vulgaris

- Papules, pustules, cysts and comedones can be seen, while the latter ones are the characteristic lesions. Comedones can be closed (white heads) or open (black heads).

- They are variably distributed and treatment is based on the lesions that are seen.

- Common areas are Face, V area of the chest, back of the trunk and upper arms. Examining all these areas could aid in the diagnosis.

- Please see Chap. 9, 'Face' for more details on its clinical presentation and management.

11.5 Atopic Dermatitis (AD)

- Atopic dermatitis is an inflammatory skin disease that is characterized by recurrent, pruritic, localized eczema, often associated with seasonal fluctuations.

- The disorder can be associated with asthma, allergic rhino conjunctivitis, food allergies and other immediate hypersensitivity allergies.

- It usually develops in childhood and may persist into adulthood; less commonly, it can start in midlife or late life.

- The clinical presentation can vary depending on age, disease stage, race or ethnic group and geographic location.

  When AD manifests on upper extremity, it usually involves flexors such as cubital fossa and ventral aspect of the wrists (Ständer 2021b) (Fig. 11.4).

  This type of presentation is more common in children above 2years and in adults.

- Please see Chap. 5, 'Eczema' for more details on its clinical presentation and management.

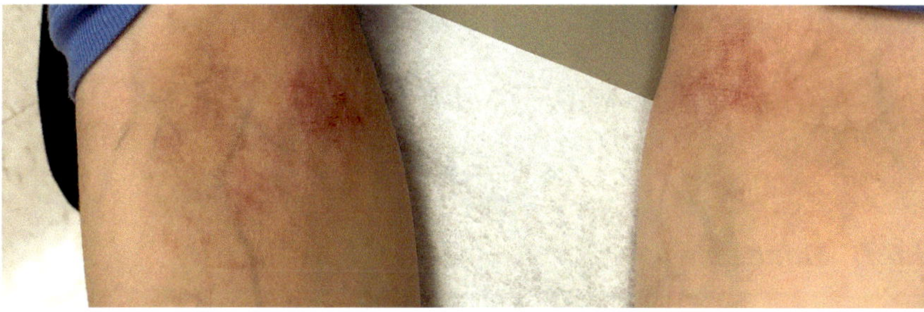

Fig. 11.4 Atopic dermatitis involving ante cubital fossa

11.6 Nummular Eczema or Nummular Dermatitis or Discoid Eczema

- Nummular eczema is characterized by intensely itchy erythematous or eczematous plaques that are oval or coin-shaped and are sharply defined (Fig. 11.5).

- Usually are multiple and bilateral in distribution.

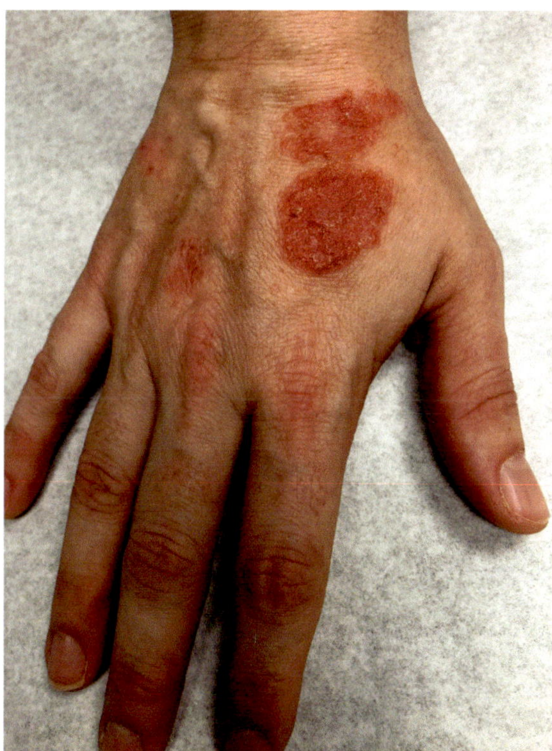

Fig. 11.5 Nummular eczema

- Common in extremities; lower limbs more than upper extremities.
- There is a large variation in size: 1 to 10cm in diameter. The lesions are usually multiple and symmetrically distributed (Leung et al. 2021).

11.6.1 Management

- Topical potent corticosteroids are usually helpful.

11.7 Psoriasis Vulgaris

- Psoriasis vulgaris is the most common type of psoriasis.
- Psoriasis vulgaris usually presents as well-demarcated, erythematous plaques with a silver scaly surface. Size is variable (Fig. 11.6).
- Common areas are extensor aspects of extremities such as back of elbow and knees, scalp and sacral area (Kessler 2022).
- Please see Chap. 3, 'Papulosqumaous Disorders' for more details on its clinical presentation and management.

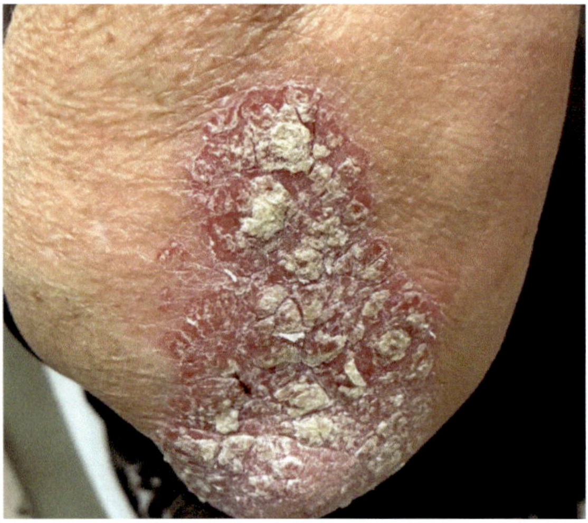

Fig. 11.6 Psoriasis vulgaris

11.8 Lichen Planus (LP)

- LP is characterized by intensely pruritic, purple, polygonal, flat-topped papules (Micheletti et al. 2023) (Fig. 11.7).

- The exact etiology of LP is unknown.

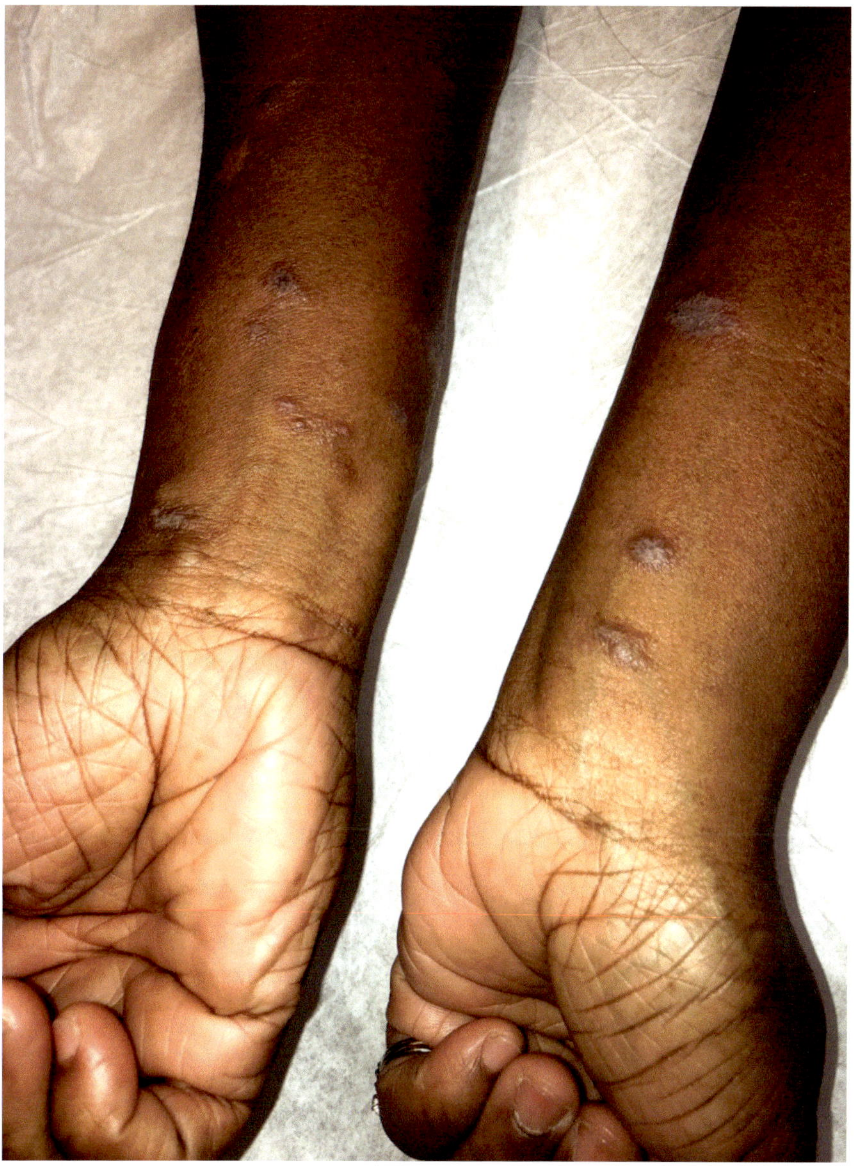

Fig. 11.7 Lichen planus

- The distribution of the eruption is symmetrical. Flexural wrists, arms and legs are common sites.

- Wickham striae characterized by white, adherent reticulate scales are characteristic of LP.

- Please see Chap. 3, 'Papulosqumaous disorders' for more details on clinical presentation, diagnosis and management of lichen planus.

Hands

- Granuloma annulare.
- Palmoplantar psoriasis.
- Pompholyx.
- Hand eczema.
- Cutaneous infections.

11.9 Granuloma Annulare (GA)

- Granuloma annulare: It is a non-infectious granulomatous disease (Wang and Khachemoune 2017).

- Several morphological forms exist. Localized, Generalized, Subcutaneous and Perforating are the common ones (Zhang et al. 2022).

- Localized is most common with classical presentation of annular shaped, skin colored or erythematous papules (Salasche 2000) (Fig. 11.8).

- Exact etiology is unknown.

- Onset more common in females below 30 years old (Muhlemann and Williams 1984).

- It has been reported to be associated with several conditions. Diabetes mellitus, thyroid disease, malignancy and hyperlipidemia are among them (Piette and Rosenbach 2016).

- Asymptomatic.

- Common sites: Dorsal hands or feet (Thornsberry and English 2013).

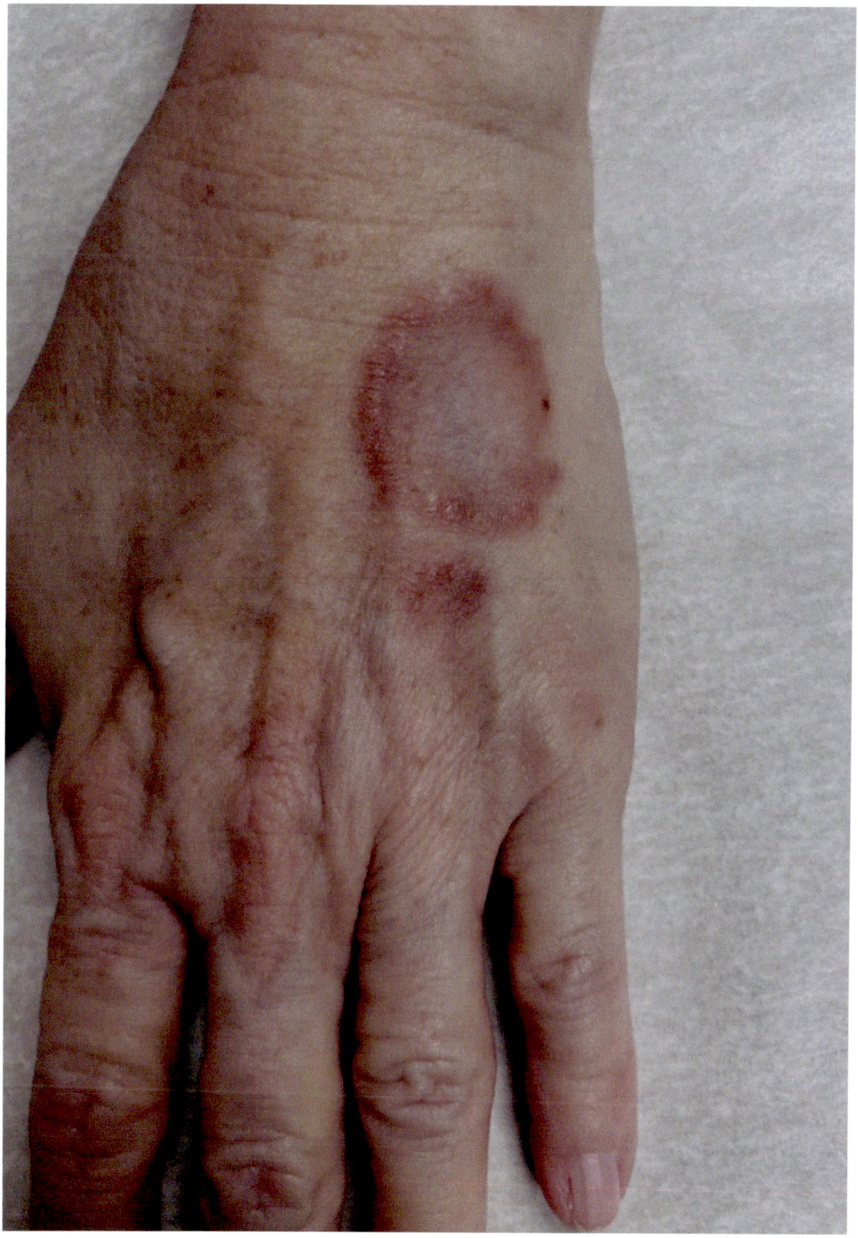

Fig. 11.8 Granuloma annualare

11.9.1 Diagnosis

- Diagnosis is usually made clinically. Tinea corporis is the main differential. Please see the chapter on cutaneous infections for its characteristic findings and that helps in differentiating both these conditions. Skin biopsy can be done if there is doubt.

11.9.2 Management

- Localized form of GA can subside on its own in 50% of the patients (Wang and Khachemoune 2017).

- Several therapeutic modalities have been in use to treat GA for those who wish to be treated. However, none of them is known to be definitely effective (Wang and Khachemoune 2017).

- Ultrapotent corticosteroids such as clobetasol propionate are usually the first line of drugs tried.

- Intralesional (IL) triamcinolone 5mg/ml have been used with success.
  - There are also reports of GA responding to IL nasal saline and also subsiding after a biopsy was done; (Kern 1960; Naveen 2014) all advocating the hypothesis that mechanical trauma may help in the resolution of GA.

- Topical tacrolimus and cryotherapy can be tried when the above measures fail (Wang and Khachemoune 2017).

- There are several other modalities that have been used with some success and cases not responding to the above measures, can be referred to dermatologist, if patient wants to be treated.

11.10 Pompholyx (Dyshydrotic Eczema)

- It is a type of endogenous eczema.

- Manifests as vesicles only on the sides of the fingers or toes (Fig. 11.9).

- Can be associated with recurrences.

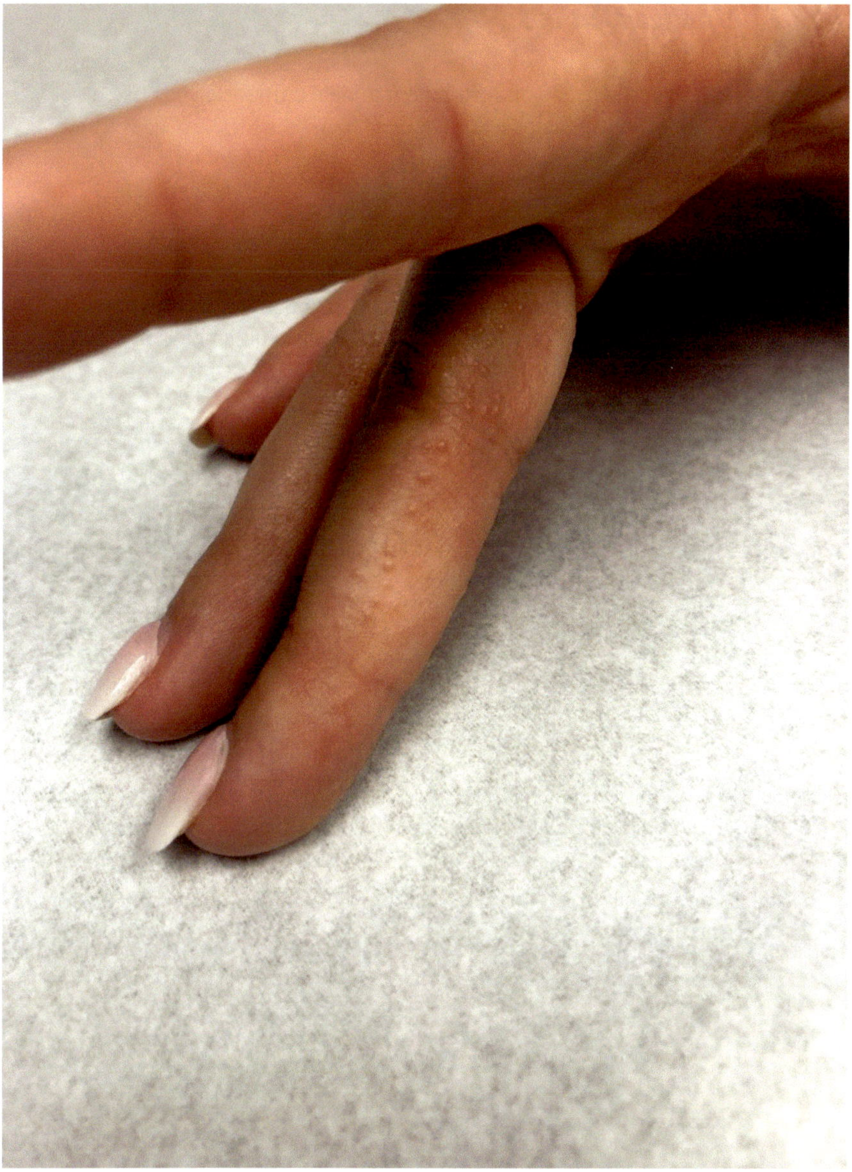

Fig. 11.9 Dyshydrotic eczema

11.10.1 Management

– Management includes usage of ultra-potent topical corticosteroids like clobetasol propionate 0.05% ointment.

11.11 Hand Eczema (Figs. 11.10 and 11.11)

– Hand eczema is usually chronic and is manifested with hyperkeratosis and fissures (Fig. 11.10). It is usually a combination of both endogenous and exogenous eczema (contact dermatitis).

– Contact dermatitis on the hands may result from the objects used in everyday use or occupational exposures.

– Given the multitude of things that come in contact with hands, often it may not be easy to pin point exactly the allergen.

– The dermatitis can be treated by ultra-potent topical steroids such as clobetasol propionate 0.05% ointment and by avoidance of the offending agent, if one is present and is identified.

– For severe chronic hand eczema refractory to potent topical corticosteroids, alitretinoin can be used (Gawkrodger and Ardern-Jones 2021).

– Often it is appropriate to refer to a dermatologist if hand eczema is not responding to topical medications.

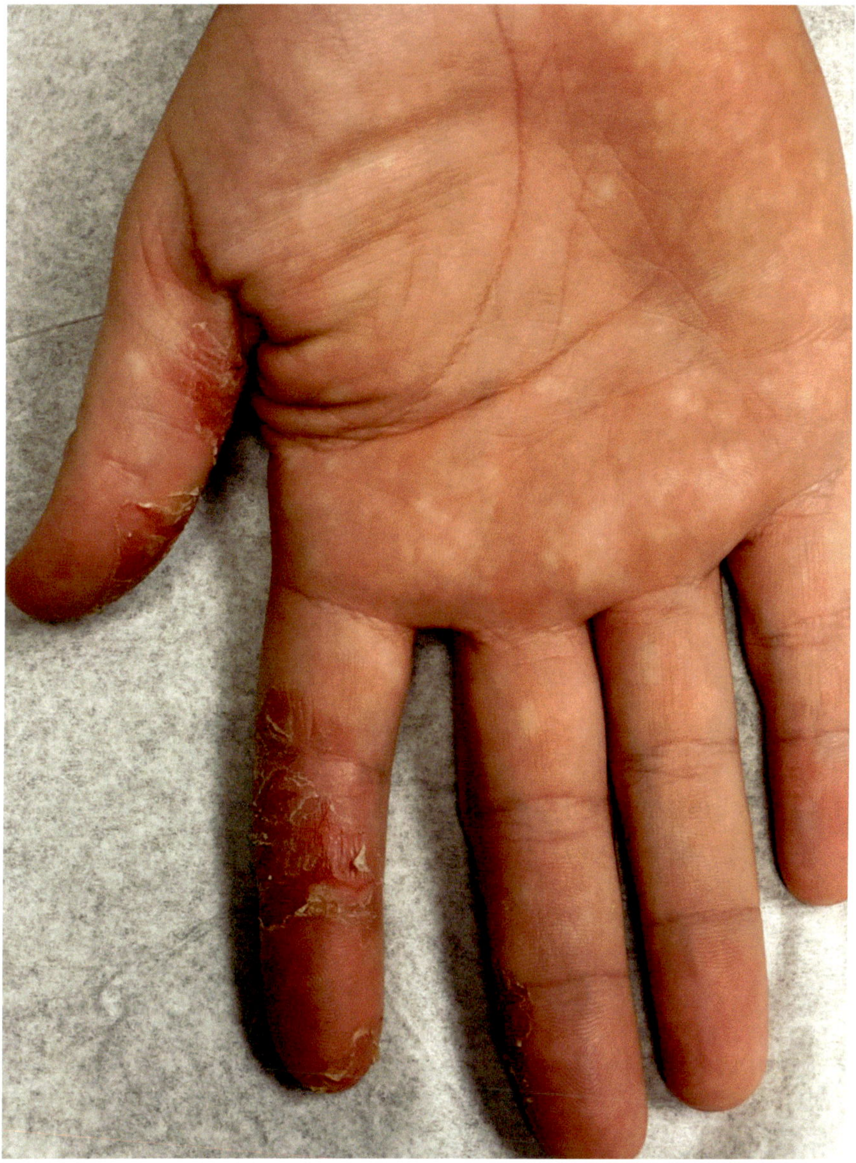

Fig. 11.10 Hand eczema involving palmar side

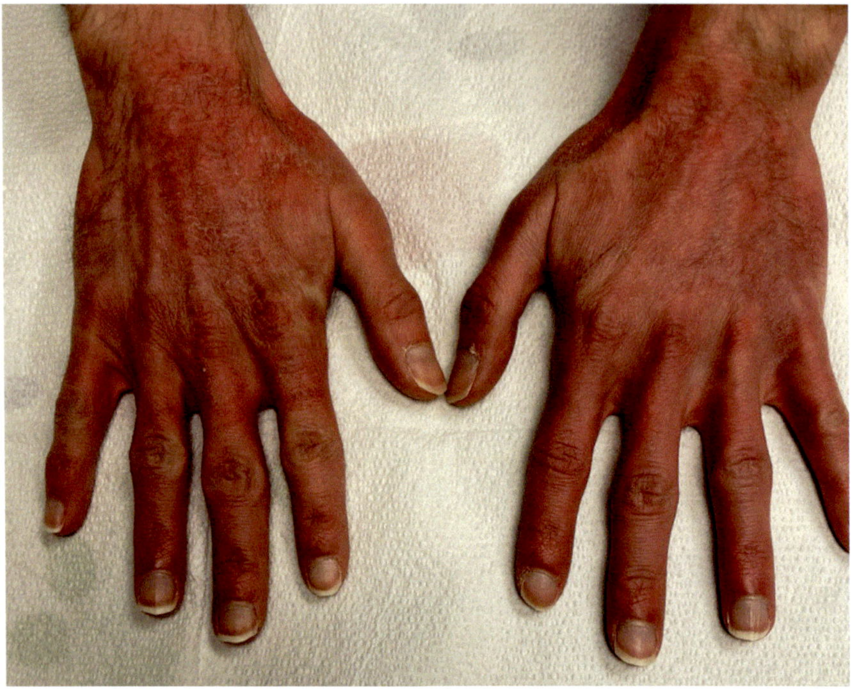

Fig. 11.11 Hand eczema manifesting on dorsal aspect

11.12 Palmoplantar Psoriasis (Figs. 11.12 and 11.13)

- Palmoplantar psoriasis is a variant of psoriasis that characteristically affects the skin of the palms and soles.
- Hyperkeratotic, pustular or mixed morphologies can occur (Engin et al. 2017).
- Hyperkeratotic is the most common one. Erythema, fissuring and scaling are noted. Itching and pain can be there.
- Usually, symmetrically distributed.

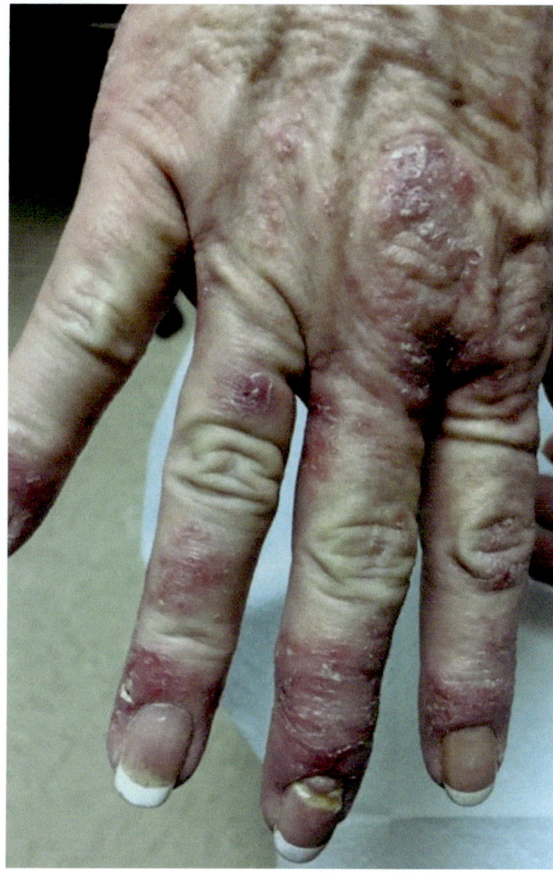

Fig. 11.12 Psoriasis hands

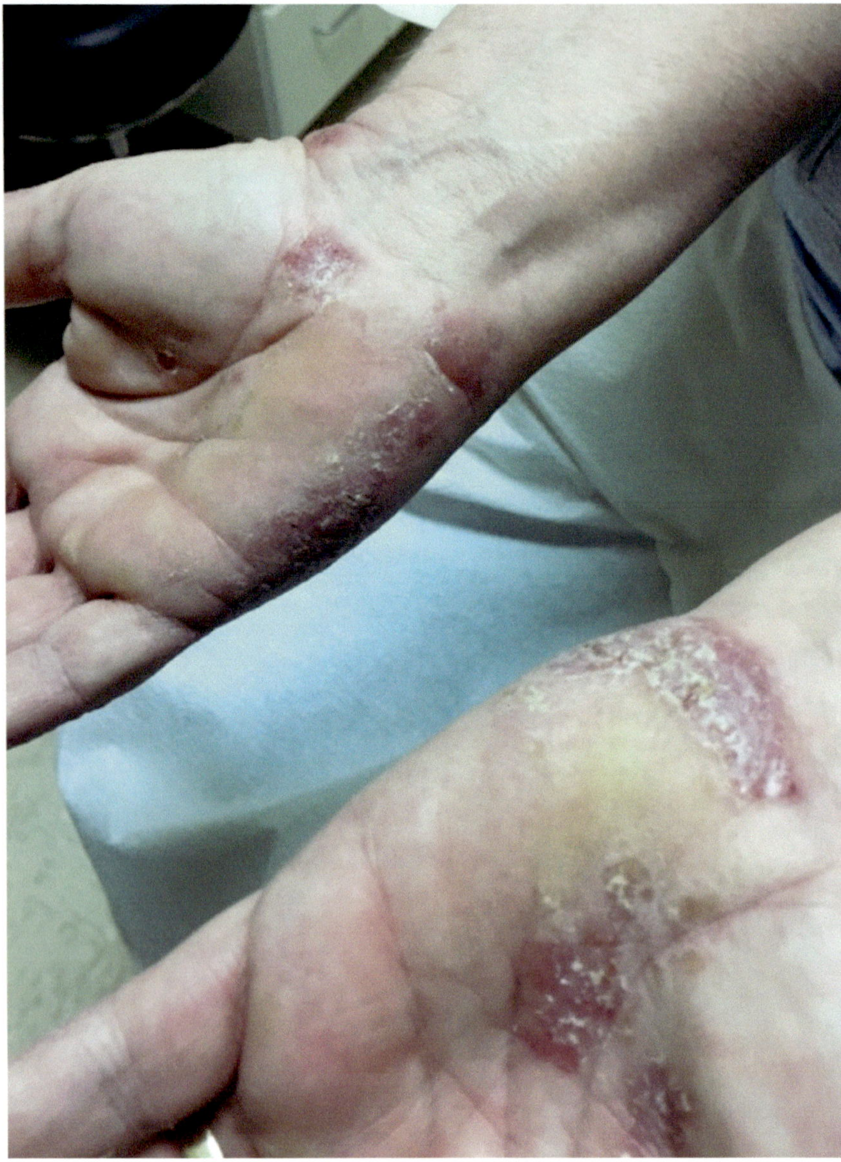

Fig. 11.13 Psoriasis palms

11.12.1 Diagnosis

- If differentiation from tinea cannot be made clinically, examination with potassium hydroxide can be done. When in doubt, skin biopsy can be done. Please see Chap. 15, 'Feet' for more details on its diagnosis.

11.12.2 Management

- Ultra (Super) potent topical corticosteroids such as clobetasol propionate 0.05% ointment applied twice daily with or without occlusion is the initial drug of choice (Engin et al. 2017).
- Calcipotriene is often combined or alternated with potent topical corticosteroids.
- Tazarotene gel applied topically is also an option.
- If not responsive to the above, referral to dermatologist may be needed to institute other treatment options such as phototherapy and systemic therapy.
- Acitretin 10–50 mg per day orally is usually the initial systemic agent used (Engin et al. 2017).
- Cyclosporine and methotrexate in doses of 7.5–20 mg weekly can be given as second line systemic agent. There are several biological drugs that can also be administered in refractory cases.
- In all patients with palmoplantar psoriatic skin disease, an assessment to diagnose any underlying joint disease should be done. If psoriatic arthritis is present, systemic therapy is warranted.

11.13 Cutaneous Infections

11.13.1 Tinea Manuum

- Please see Chap. 6, 'Common Cutaneous Infections' for details on its clinical presentation, diagnosis and management.

11.13.2 Acute Staphylococcal Paronychia

- Cellulitis of the proximal nail fold (Fig. 11.14).

- **Management:** Incision and drainage to be done and the discharge is to be sent for culture and sensitivity. Treatment as per culture and sensitivity. While waiting on the culture, if MRSA is suspected clindamycin or Trimethoprim-sulfamethoxazole are the common drugs that are preferred. For MSSA, Cephalexin or dicloxacillin can be given.

- Other cutaneous infections described in Chap. 6, 'Common Cutaneous Infections' can also occur on upper extremity and hands.

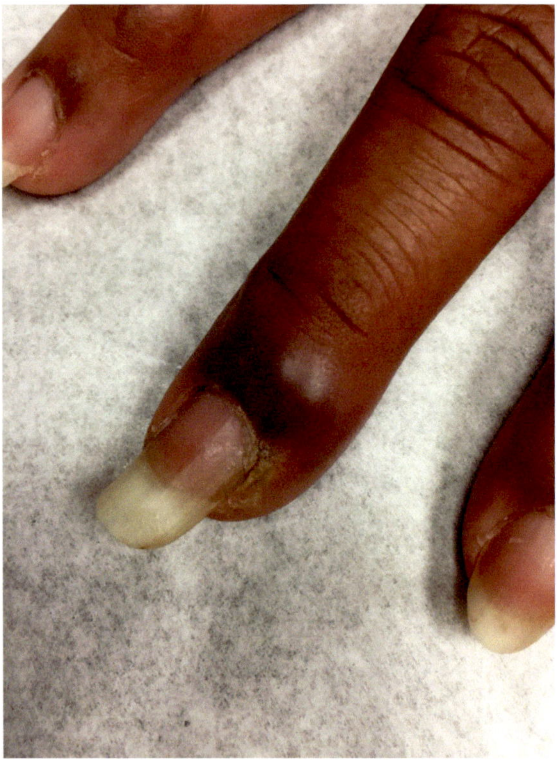

Fig. 11.14 Acute paronychia

Bibliography

Berman B, Cockerell CJ. Pathobiology of actinic keratosis: ultraviolet-dependent keratinocyte proliferation. J Am Acad Dermatol. 2013;68(1):S10–9.

Bruckner AL. Keratosis pilaris and other follicular keratotic disorders. In: Kang S, Amagai M, Bruckner AL, Enk AH, Margolis DJ, McMichael AJ, Orringer JS, editors. Fitzpatrick's dermatology. Vol. 9e. McGraw-Hill Education; 2019

Cho SI, Kim JW, Yeo G, Choi D, Seo J, Yoon HS, et al. Senile purpura: clinical features and related factors. Ann Dermatol. 2019;31(4):472–5. https://www.ncbi.nlm.nih.gov/pmc/articles/PMC7992766/

Cohen L, Seminario-Vidal L, Lockey RF. Dermatologic problems commonly seen by the allergist/immunologist. J Allergy Clin Immunol. 2020;8(1):102–12

Criscione VD, Weinstock MA, Naylor MF, Luque C, Eide MJ, Bingham SF. Actinic keratoses. Cancer. 2009;115(11):2523–30.

Czarnecki D, Meehan CJ, Bruce F, Culjak G. The majority of cutaneous squamous cell carcinomas arise in actinic keratoses. JCMS. 2002;6(3):207–9.

Eisen DB, Asgari MM, Bennett DD, Connolly SM, Dellavalle RP, Freeman EE, et al. Guidelines of care for the management of actinic keratosis. J Am Acad Dermatol. 2021;0(0). https://www.jaad.org/article/S0190-9622(21)00502-8/fulltext

Engin B, Aşkın Ö, Tüzün Y. Palmoplantar psoriasis. Clin Dermatol. 2017;35(1):19–27.

Elmets CA, Viner JL, Pentland AP, Cantrell W, Lin HY, Bailey H, et al. Chemoprevention of nonmelanoma skin cancer with celecoxib: a randomized, double-blind, placebo-controlled trial. JNCI. 2010;102(24):1835–44

Fenske NA, Lober CW. Structural and functional changes of normal aging skin. J Am Acad Dermatol. 1986;15(4):571–85.

Gawkrodger DJ, Ardern-Jones MR. Dermatology: an illustrated colour text. London: Elsevier; 2021.

Gerbig AW. Treating keratosis pilaris. J Am Acad Dermatol. 2002;47(3):457–67.

Glogau RG. The risk of progression to invasive disease. J Am Acad Dermatol. 2000;42(1):S23–4.

Hosking AM, Elsensohn A, Makdisi J, Grando S, Sebastien de Feraudy. Keratosis pilaris rubra with mucin deposition. J Cutan Pathol. 2018;45(12):958–61

Kessler TR. Treating patients with moderate-to-severe psoriasis vulgaris. J Am Acad Phys Assis. 2022 (Publish Ahead of Print)

Kern AB. Injection therapy of granuloma annulare. Arch Dermatol. 1960;81(6):969–9

Kerns ML, Chien AL, Kang S. Skin aging. In: Kang S, Amagai M, Bruckner AL, Enk AH, Margolis DJ, McMichael AJ, Orringer JS. editors. Fitzpatrick's dermatology. Vol. 9e. McGraw-Hill Education; 2019

Leonard HG, Mamelak AJ. Review ofactinic keratosis. Part I: etiology, epidemiology and clinical presentation. PubMed. 2010;9(9):1125–32

Leung AKC, Lam JM, Leong KF, Leung AAM, Wong AHC, Hon KL. Nummular eczema: an updated review. Recent Pat Inflam Allergy Drug Discov. 2021;14(2):146–55.

Marks R, Foley P, Goodman G, Hage BH, Selwood TS. Spontaneous remission of solar keratoses: the case for conservative management. Br J Dermatol. 1986;115(6):649–55

Marks R, Rennie G, Selwood Thomas S. Malignant transformation of solar keratoses to squamous cell carcinoma. Lancet. 1988;331(8589):795–7

Micheletti RG, James WD, Elston DM, McMahon PJ. Andrews' diseases of the skin: clinical atlas. St. Louis, Missouri: Elsevier; 2023.

Mittelbronn MA, Mullins DL, Ramos-Caro FA, Flowers FP. Frequency of pre-existing actinic keratosis in cutaneous squamous cell carcinoma. Int J Dermatol. 1998;37(9):677–81.

Muhlemann MF, Williams DRR. Localized granuloma annulare is associated with insulin-dependent diabetes mellitus. Br J Dermatol. 1984;111(3):325–9.

Naveen K, Pai VV, Athanikar SB, Gupta G, Parshwanath HA. Remote reverse Koebner phenomenon in generalized granuloma annulare. 2014;5(2):219–9

Pennycook KB, McCready TA. Keratosis pilaris. In: StatPearls. Treasure Island (FL): StatPearls Publishing; 2024. PMID: 31536314

Piette EW, Rosenbach M. Granuloma annulare: Pathogenesis, disease associations and triggers, and therapeutic options. J Am Acad Dermatol. 2016;75(3):467–79. https://pubmed.ncbi.nlm.nih.gov/27543210/

Salasche SJ. Epidemiology of actinic keratoses and squamous cell carcinoma. J Am Acad Dermatol. 2000;42(1):S4-7.

Ständer S. Atopic dermatitis. New Eng J Med. 2021;384(12):1136–43 (Ropper AH, editor)

Thornsberry LA, English JC. Etiology, diagnosis, and therapeutic management of granuloma annulare: an update. Am J Clin Dermatol. 2013;14(4):279–90.

Wang J, Khachemoune A. Granuloma annulare: a focused review of therapeutic options. Am J Clin Dermatol. 2017;19(3):333–44.

Werner RN, Sammain A, Erdmann R, Hartmann V, Stockfleth E, Nast A. The natural history of actinic keratosis: a systematic review. Br J Dermatol. 2013;169(3):502–18.

Zhang L, Jiang C, Wang W, He L, Chen T. Auricular granuloma annulare. Indian J Dermatol Venereol Leprol. 2022;17:1–4.

Chapter 12
Axilla

Abstract There are relatively few common dermatological conditions that involve axilla. This chapter provides an overview of those common skin conditions. The chapter discusses mainly from their clinical perspective. It provides details about the clinical presentation of these conditions and ways to diagnose them; where feasible, it provides clinical information regarding how to diagnose them clinically. It also discusses their treatment options and when appropriate the circumstances as to when the patients need to be referred to the dermatologist.

Keywords Contact dermatitis · Tinea axillaries · Candidiasis · Erythrasma · Hidradenitis suppurative · Tinea

12.1 Contact Dermatitis

- Contact dermatitis needs to be always ruled out in any rashes in the axilla. Please see if there is any history of recent change in deodorants (the common culprits). While the positive history could make a diagnosis of contact Dermatitis more likely, absence of that history does not rule out completely contact dermatitis.

- Often the 'Stick' or 'bar' type of deodorant causes folliculitis type of contact dermatitis (Fig. 12.1) while the spray type cause erythematous patches (Fig. 12.2).

- The rash due to contact dermatitis can be unilateral or bilateral.

- **Treatment** includes stopping the suspected deodorant and prescribing topical moderately potent steroid or potent steroid depending on the intensity of the inflammation.
  - If it is found that patient has been using the stick or bar type of deodorant changing that to spray type could help.

D. K. Yellumahanthi, *Manual of Primary Care Dermatology*,
https://doi.org/10.1007/978-3-031-68406-7_12

– Often fragrance in the deodorant is a potential allergen. If despite using fragrance free deodorant, if the rash comes back, patch testing may be necessary to precisely advise the patient regarding what deodorant to use. A referral to a dermatologist is appropriate at that time.

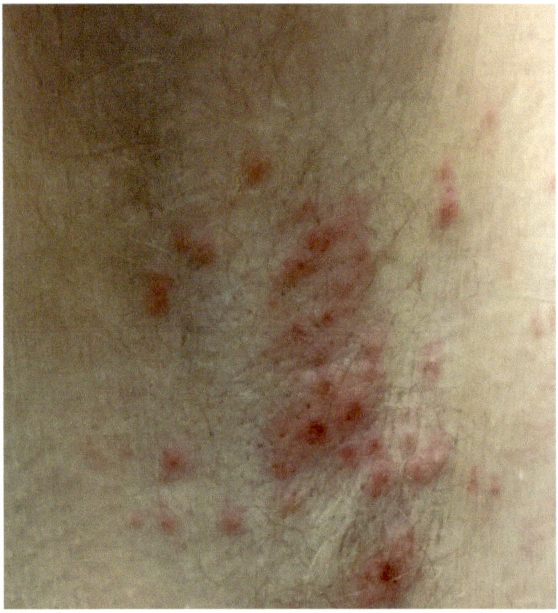

Fig. 12.1 Folliculitis type of contact dermatitis secondary to use of stick type of deodorant

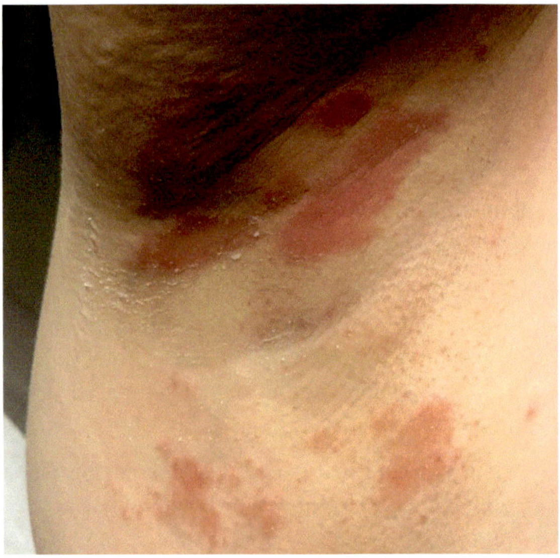

Fig. 12.2 Patch type of contact dermatitis secondary to use of spray type of deodorant

12.2 Cutaneous Infections

12.2.1 Tinea Axillaris (Fig. 12.3)

- Caused by fungi known as dermatophytes.

- Usually presents as erythematous plaque. Unlike the lesions of contact dermatitis, the lesions of tinea axillaris show central clearing. The borders are raised and faint scaling can be noticed.

- **Diagnosis:** Examination with potassium hydroxide (KOH) can be performed in the office to confirm the diagnosis. A culture for fungus & a skin biopsy for histo pathological examination can also be done.

- **Treatment:** Topical imidazoles such as clotrimazole, miconazole, ketoconazole or allylamines (terbinafine) can be used.

- Oral terbinafine or fluconazole can also be used if topical treatment is not effective in adults (Craddock and Schieke 2019).

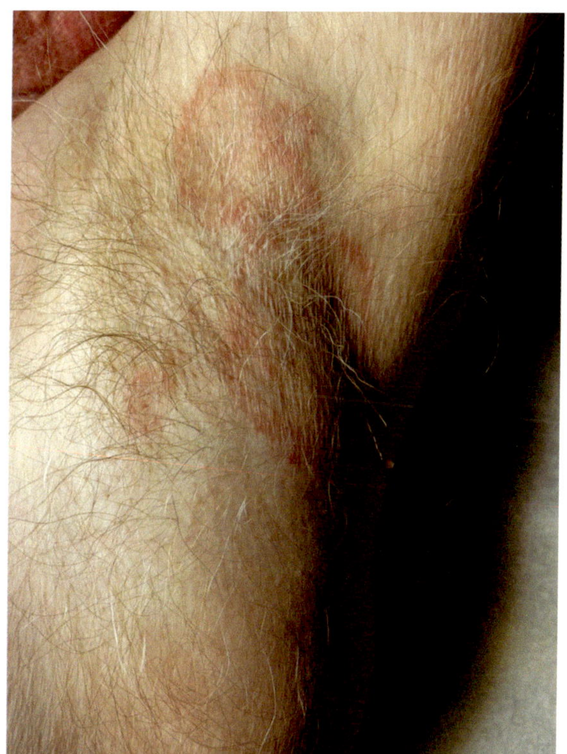

Fig. 12.3 Tinea axillaris

12.2.2 *Candidiasis*

– Erythematous patches that may look moist or macerated. Satellite lesions are usually seen (Fig. 12.4). Diagnosis can be made based on the clinical appearance. When in doubt, potassium hydroxide preparation can aid in the diagnosis.

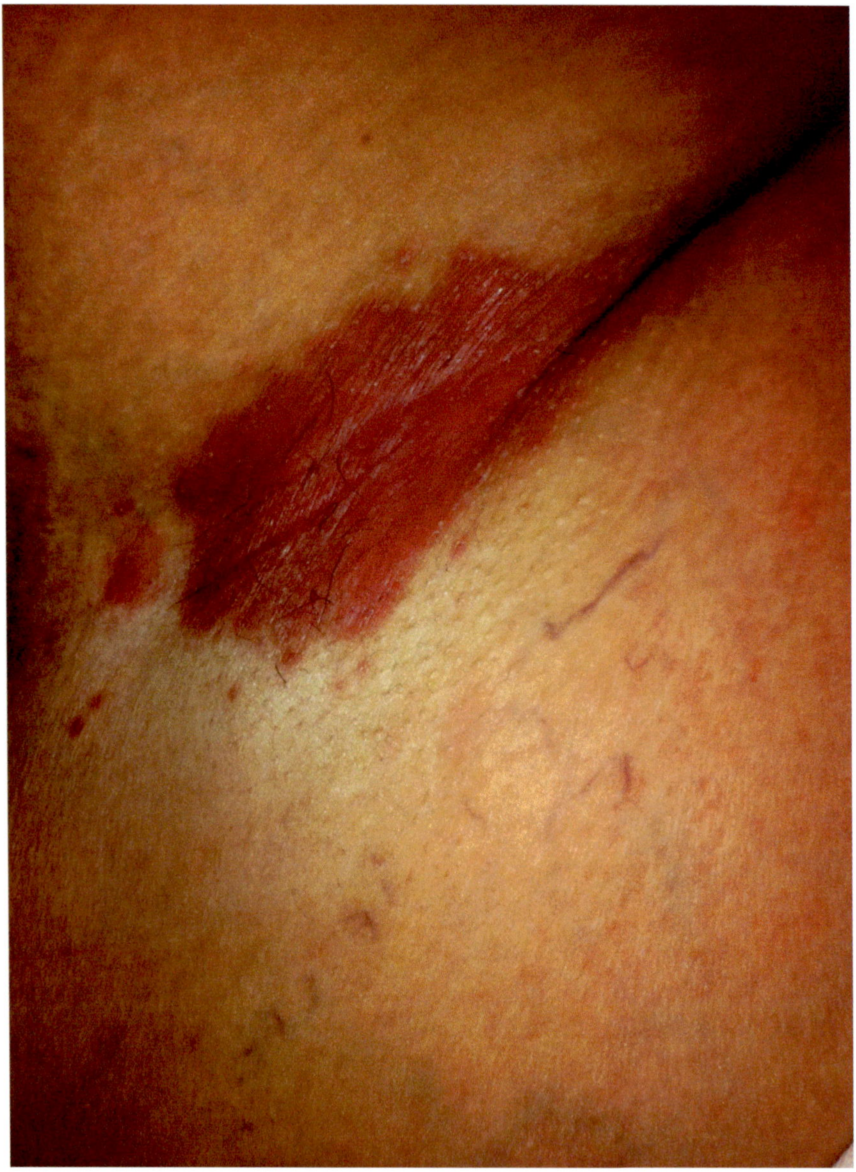

Fig. 12.4 Candidiasis

– **Treatment:** Topical antifungals: Nystatin or imidazoles such as clotrimazole, miconazole, ketoconazole can be used.

  Oral antifungals: Fluconazole, or Itraconazole can be used if refractory to topical agents (Taudorf et al. 2019).

12.2.3 Erythrasma (Fig. 12.5)

– The etiologic agent is *Corynebacterium minutissimum.*

– Please see Chap. 6, 'Common Cutaneous Infections' for details on clinical presentation, diagnosis and management of erythrasma.

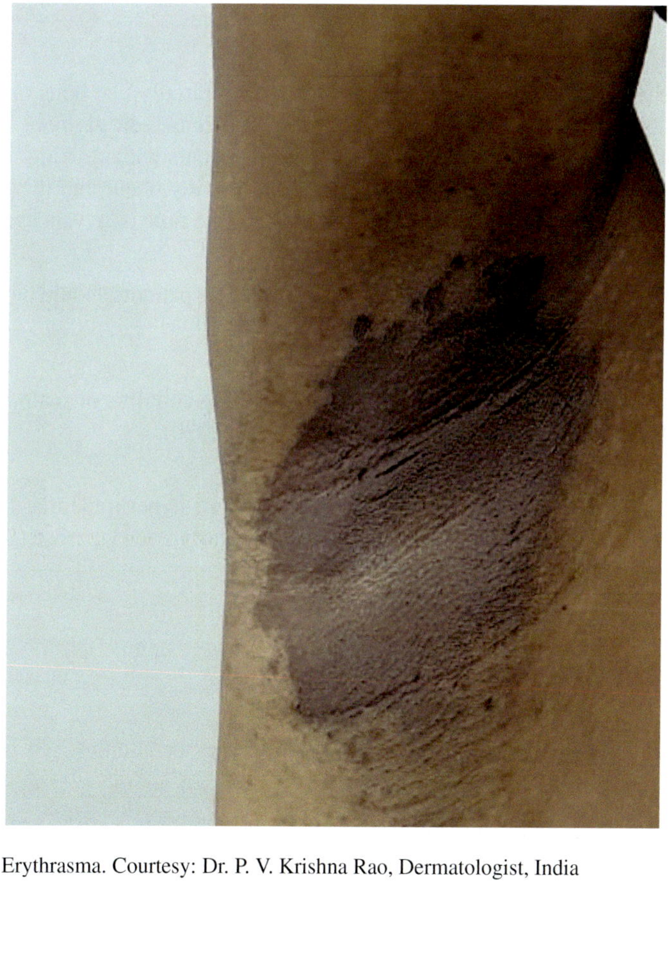

Fig. 12.5 Erythrasma. Courtesy: Dr. P. V. Krishna Rao, Dermatologist, India

12.3 Hidradenitis Suppurativa (HS)

- Hidradenitis suppurativa (HS) is a chronic inflammatory disorder of the hair follicles in intertrigionous areas such as axilla, inframammary folds, groins and anogenital regions of the body.

- Usually more than one site is involved.

- Manifests initially after puberty. More common in females.

- The pathogenesis of HS is multifactorial. Genetic susceptibility, hormone dysregulation and hair follicle occlusion are among them (Jenkins et al. 2023).

- The clinical presentation is characterized by recurrent painful nodules, sinus tracts and long term sequel such as scarring and contractures.

- The early manifestations are abscesses that appear initially like boils or nodules. These abscesses if not treated can break open and cause seropurulent discharge and can lead to chronic draining sinuses. Healing occurs with scarring. However, complete healing of resolving abscesses do not usually occur and there may be some constant little drainage and inflammation all the time (Gavvala et al. 2013).

- HS can be associated with several conditions and thus patients should be screened for all potential conditions that can be associated.

- It can be associated with acne conglobata, dissecting cellulitis of scalp, pilonidal sinus (follicular occlusion tetrad) (Goldburg et al. 2020).

- Patients also need to be screened for hypertension, hyperlipidemia, metabolic syndrome, polycystic ovarian syndrome, inflammatory bowel disease (Shlyankevich et al. 2014).

12.3.1 Management

- **Mild cases:** Isolated solitary or multiple abscesses or nodules. No tunnels or scarring.
  - Topical clindamycin with oral tetracyclines is the common regimen employed. Oral antibiotics are tried for about 4 months. Topical metronidazole 0.75% gel and topical erythromycin can be used as alternatives to clindamycin.

Macrolides, trimethoprim-sulfamethoxazole, ampicillin and cephalexin can be used when tetracyclines cannot be given.

- In refractory cases, clindamycin 300mg with Rifampin 300mg orally can be given 2–3 times daily in adult patients (Gao and Acne 2022).
- Intralesional triamcinolone therapy can be effective for isolated HS lesions (Shanmugam et al. 2017).

- **Moderate** (Fig. 12.6): Single or multiple abscesses that are apart. One or more Sinus tracts and scarring present.
  - In addition to the above therapy, tumor necrosis factor alfa inhibitors are effective and safe for the treatment of HS; Adalimumab is approved by the US Food and Drug Administration for HS (Goldburg et al. 2019).

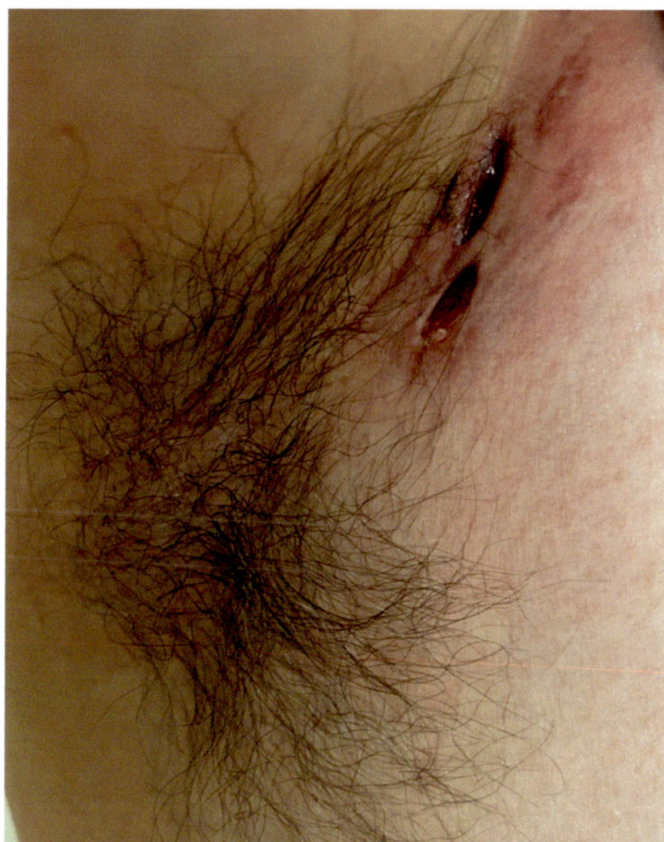

Fig. 12.6 Moderate HS with sinus tracts and scarring

- **Severe:** (Fig. 12.8) Diffuse involvement with multiple interconnected sinus tracts and abscesses.
  - Usually requires surgical intervention or laser therapy.
  - In general, only mild HS (Fig. 12.7) has scope to be managed in primary care. If HS is not responding to antibiotic therapy, it may be prudent to refer to dermatology for further management (Fig. 12.8).

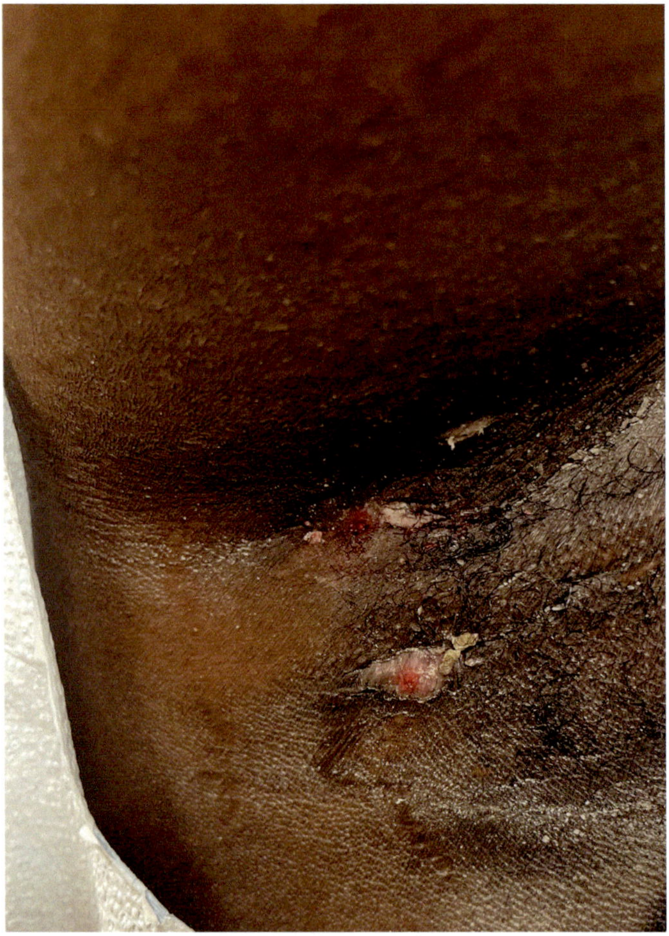

Fig. 12.7 Mild HS with isolated lesions with no sinus tracts or scarring

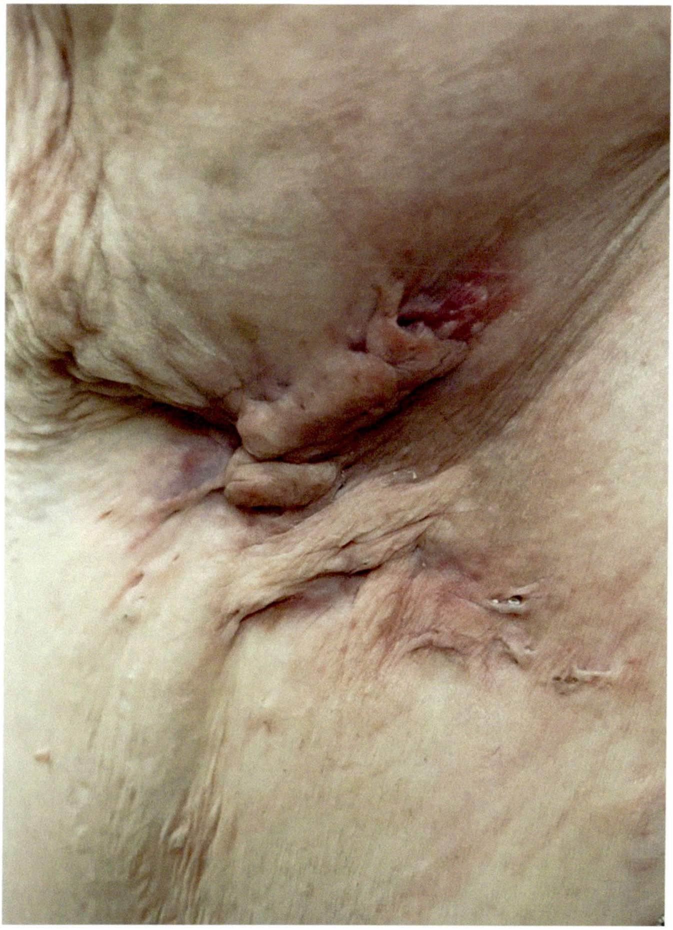

Fig. 12.8 HS with extensive and confluent lesions and scarring

Bibliography

Craddock LN, Schieke SM. Superficial fungal infection. In: Kang S, Amagai M, Bruckner AL, Enk AH, Margolis DJ, McMichael AJ, Orringer JS, editors. Fitzpatrick's dermatology. Vol 9e. 2019

Gao Y, Acne FR, Rosacea, and related disorders. In: Soutor C, Hordinsky MK. Editors. Clinical dermatology: diagnosis and management of common disorders, Vol 2e. McGraw-Hill Education; 2022

Gavvala M, Waseem B, Nina N. Disorders of sweat glands In: Sacchidanand S, Oberoi C, Inamadar A, editors. IADVL textbook of dermatology. 4th edn. Wiley; 2013

Goldburg SR, Strober BE, Payette MJ. Hidradenitis suppurativa. J Am Acad Dermatol. 2020;82(5):1045–58.

Goldburg SR, Strober BE, Payette MJ. Part 2. Current and emerging treatments for hidradenitis suppurativa. J Am Acad Dermatol. 2019

Jenkins T, Isaac J, Edwards A, Okoye GA. Hidradenitis Suppurativa. Dermatol Clin. 2023. https://www.nottsapc.nhs.uk/media/1863/hidradenitis-suppurativa.pdf

Shanmugam VK, Zaman NM, McNish S, Hant FN. Review of Current Immunologic Therapies for Hidradenitis Suppurativa. Int J Rheumatol. 2017;2017:1–6.

Shlyankevich J, Chen AJ, Kim MO, Kimball AB. Hidradenitis suppurativa is a systemic disease with substantial comorbidity burden: a chart-verified case-control analysis. J Am Acad Dermatol. 2014;71(6):1144–50.

Taudorf EH, Jemec GBE, Hay RJ, Saunte DML. Cutaneous candidiasis—an evidence-based review of topical and systemic treatments to inform clinical practice. J Eur Acad Dermatol Venereol JEADV. 2019;33(10):1863–73. https://pubmed.ncbi.nlm.nih.gov/31287594/

Chapter 13
Genitals and Groin

Abstract This chapter provides an overview of the common dermatological conditions such as tinea cruris, erythrasma, candidiasis, flexural psoriasis, lichen sclerosus et atrophicus that can involve genital and groin area. The chapter discusses mainly from their clinical perspective. It provides details about the clinical presentation of these conditions and ways to diagnose them; where appropriate it provides clinical information regarding how to diagnose them clinically. It also discusses their treatment options and where appropriate the circumstances as to when the patients need to be referred to the dermatologist.

Keywords Tinea cruris · Erythrasma · Candidiasis · Flexural psoriasis · Lichen sclerosus et atrophicus · Pearly papules of penis · Warts · Herpes

13.1 Tinea Cruris

- Manifests as bright red annular plaques that affect the lateral and medial groin folds. The borders are usually raised (Fig. 13.1).

- Buttocks could be involved. Usually, spares the scrotum, penis and female genitalia.

- There could be fine scaling.

- Itching is present.

- Usually bilateral.

D. K. Yellumahanthi, *Manual of Primary Care Dermatology*,
https://doi.org/10.1007/978-3-031-68406-7_13

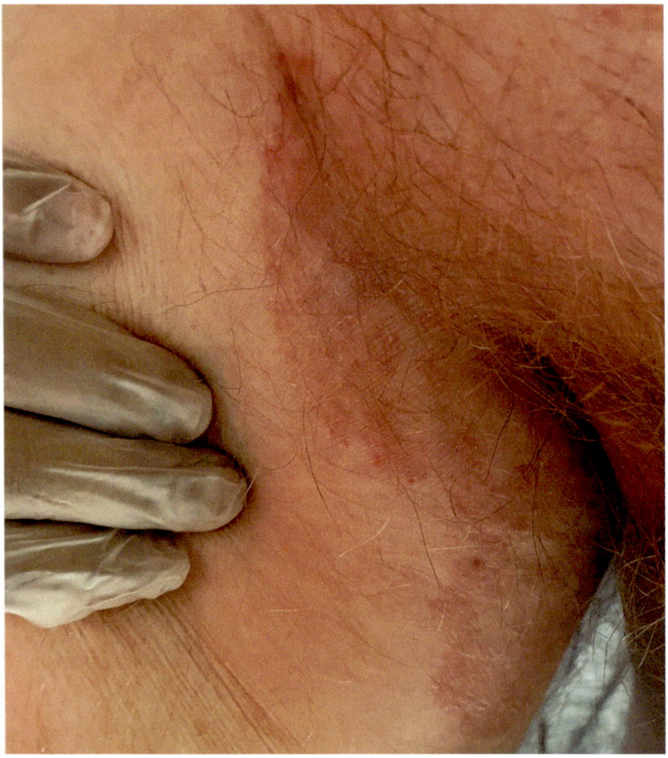

Fig. 13.1 Tinea cruris

13.1.1 Diagnosis

– A potassium hydroxide (KOH) prep can be performed in the office to confirm the diagnosis. A culture for fungus and skin biopsy can also be done to confirm the diagnosis as well.

13.1.2 Management

– Topical antifungals should help in most cases. For instance, topical clotrimazole, miconazole, ketoconazole, terbinafine and ciclopirox can be used.

– Oral terbinafine daily (250 mg for adults) for two weeks, fluconazole 150 mg orally weekly for four weeks can also be used if topical treatment is not effective (Craddock and Schieke 2019).

– Please see Chap. 6, 'Common Cutaneous Infections' for more details on its clinical presentation and management.

13.2 Erythrasma

- Erythrasma is manifested by well-defined but irregular reddish-brown patches, occurring in the intertriginous areas (Fig. 13.2).

- Mostly asymptomatic or causes minimal itching.

- It can be differentiated from T. cruris by clinical features such as the absence of scaling and absence of raised borders.

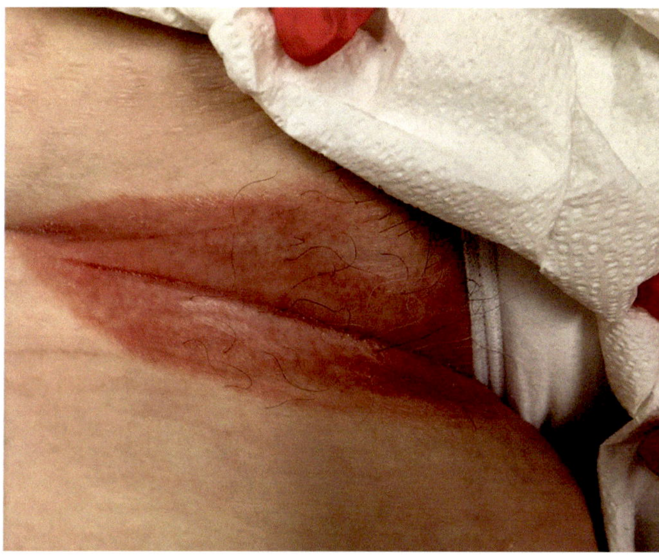

Fig. 13.2 Erythrasma

13.2.1 Management

- Treatment includes azole creams, topical clindamycin or erythromycin. Benzoyl peroxide 5% gel is also effective in most scenarios. For cases not responding to topical therapy, a 2-week course of oral erythromycin 250 mg orally four times a day, is effective in adults. A single dose of 1gm clarithromycin is an alternative. Oral tetracycline is also effective (Blaise et al. 2008; Holdiness 2002).

- Please see Chap. 6, 'Common Cutaneous Infections' for more details on its clinical presentation and management.

13.3 Candidiasis

- It manifests as bright red erythematous, moist papules, patches and plaques.

- It tends to involve body folds as well as convex surfaces.

- Satellite lesions in the form of papules and pustules are frequently observed.

- In uncircumcised men, it most commonly occurs on the glans and corona and presents as fissures at the tip of the prepuce (Fig. 13.3).

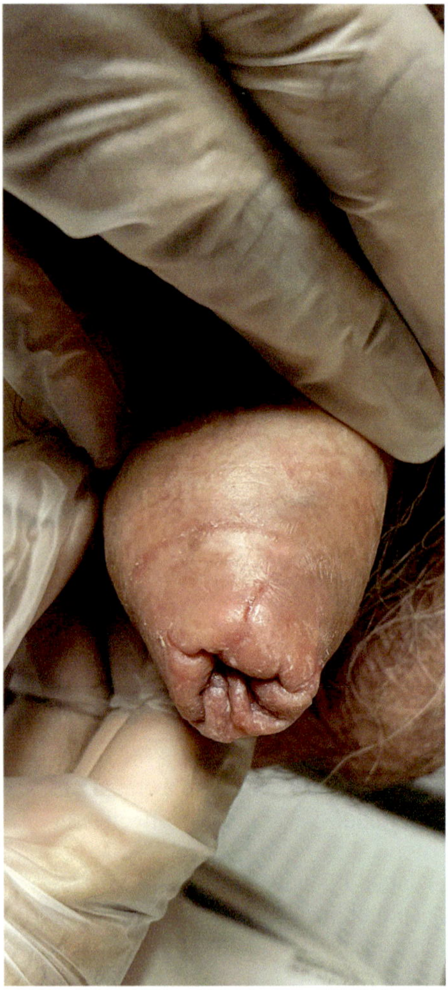

Fig. 13.3 Candida balanitis manifesting as fissures at the tip of the penis

13.3.1 *Management*

- Topical antifungals Nystatin, imidazole or azole cream or powder can be used.
- Oral fluconazole or itraconazole can be used if refractory to topical agents (Taudorf et al. 2019).
- Please see Chap. 6, 'Common Cutaneous Infections' for more details on its clinical presentation and management.

13.4 Contact Dermatitis

- Both irritant contact dermatitis and allergic contact dermatitis can occur.
- Irritant contact dermatitis is acute. The list of common irritants includes feces, urine, sweat, bathing products such as soaps, lubricants and menstrual products (O'Gorman and Torgerson 2013).
- In the acute scenario, symptoms may include erythema, edema, vesicles and ulcerations. Mild cases may manifest only with mild erythema or just stinging/burning without any skin manifestations (Shumway 2022).
- In contrast to irritant contact dermatitis, the symptoms of allergic contact dermatitis are not very pronounced and detailed history of all the items that can come in contact and can cause dermatitis needs to be ruled out.

13.4.1 *Diagnosis*

- When all the symptoms of erythema, edema and vesicles are present, the diagnosis is often obvious. If only erythema is present, if common dermatosis described above (Tinea cruris, erythrasma, candidia) are ruled out, consider contact dermatitis before any referral is made.

13.4.2 *Management*

- Like in any contact dermatitis scenario, the offending agent needs to be identified and avoided. Depending upon the extent of inflammation, topical steroids need to given. Low potent steroids for mild inflammation and moderately potent ones if inflammation is severe.

13.5 Inverse or Flexural Psoriasis

- Although psoriasis classically affects extensor aspects, at times, psoriatic lesions may be localized to the major skin folds. For instance, axilla and the genitocrural region. When it occurs in these areas, it is called as inverse or flexural psoriasis. Unlike the traditional psoriatic lesions, scaling is usually minimal or absent in flexural psoriasis (Fig. 13.4).

- The lesions show erythema that is glossy and sharply demarcated (beefy red) (Gudjonsson and Elder 2019).

- Genital psoriasis, in men, commonly affects the shaft of the penis and scrotum are common sites. In women, labia majora and perineum are the common areas of involvement (Shumway 2022).

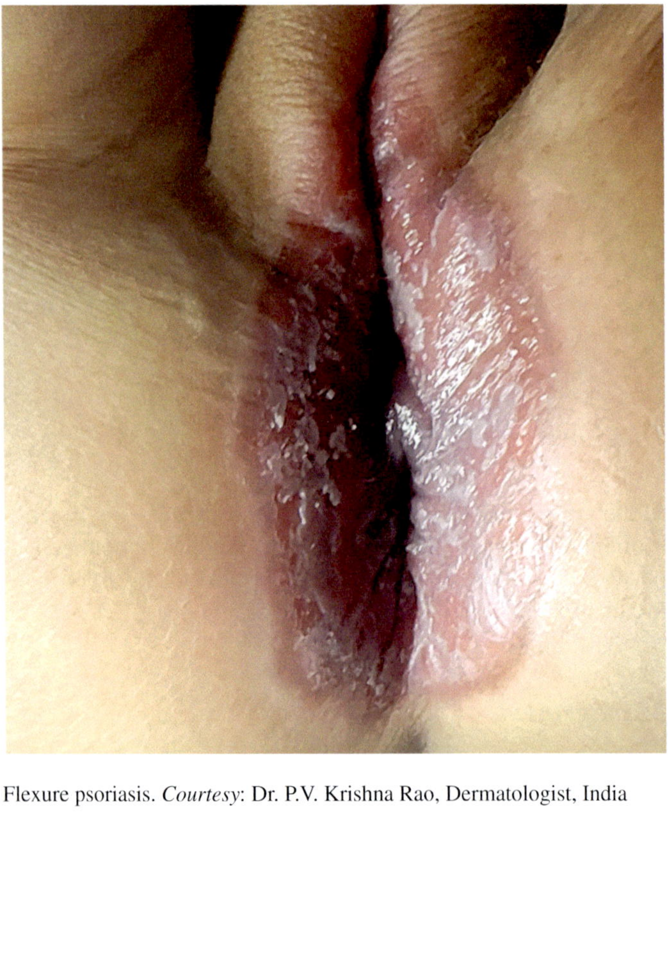

Fig. 13.4 Flexure psoriasis. *Courtesy*: Dr. P.V. Krishna Rao, Dermatologist, India

– Given that sole involvement of genital region is not all that common, when attempting to make a diagnosis of genital psoriasis, a thorough examination of all the common areas of involvement of psoriasis such as scalp, back of the elbows and knees, gluteal cleft and nails for signs of psoriasis should be made. Psoriatic arthritis also needs to be ruled out.

13.5.1 Diagnosis

– Diagnosis of Flexural psoriasis is usually based on clinical examination. If clinical examination and history are not helpful to establish the diagnosis, skin biopsy can be done.

13.5.2 Management

– Low-potency topical corticosteroids such as desonide 0.05% cream, vitamin D3 analogues (calcipotriene) and calcineurin inhibitors such as tacrolimus 0.1% ointment or pimecrolimus 1% are first choice treatments (van de Kerkhof et al. 2007).

13.6 Lichen Sclerosus et Atrophicus

– Three to ten times more common in women (Kirtschig 2016).

– Pruritus, burning; pain with ulceration are the usual symptoms. Dysuria and dyspareunia can also occur.

– On examination, erythema, with or without hypopigmentation is noticed in early stages. When hypopigmented patches occur, they are usually around the vulva and anus in the shape of 'figure of eight'.

– Typical ivory white macules and plaques are noticed in the late stages. May obstruct urethral orifice. Can cause phimosis in boys.

– Over a period of time, invasive squamous cell cancer can arise at the affected sites.

13.6.1 Diagnosis

- Often the diagnosis is made clinically based on clinical presentation. Skin biopsy can be done to confirm the diagnosis in cases where diagnosis is not certain clinically.

13.6.2 Management

- The recommended initial treatment of lichen sclerosus is application of potent to super potent topical corticosteroids such as clobetasol ointment. Calcineurin inhibitors (tacrolimus and pimecrolimus) are next line of treatment options (Kirtschig 2016). While these are not as efficacious as topical ultrapotent steroids, they do not have the side effects that can come with the topical steroids.

13.7 Pearly Penile Papules

- They are skin colored papules that are dome shaped and asymptomatic and are seen along the corona of glans penis (Fig. 13.5).

- Usually 1–2 mm in size.

- They are known to be related to angiofibromas structurally (Honigman et al. 2019).

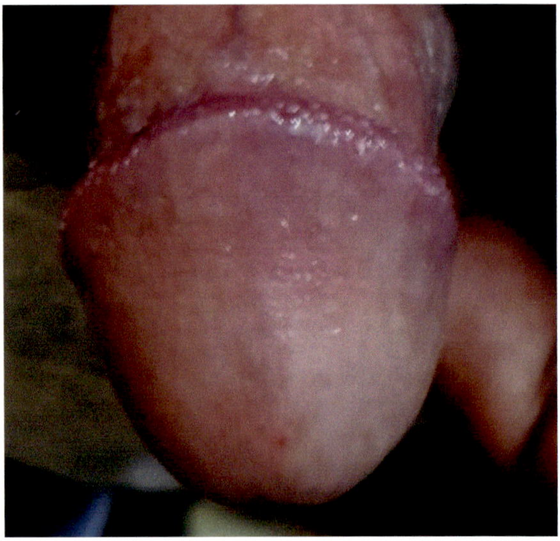

Fig. 13.5 Pearly penile papules along the corona sulcus. *Courtesy*: Dr. P.V. Krishna Rao, Dermatologist, India

13.7.1 Management

- Reassurance to the patient.

13.8 Genital Warts (Fig. 13.6)

- They can manifest with wide range of sizes. They could present as papules that are barely visible to nodules to confluent masses.

- They can be skin colored or pink or black or brown or red.

- Asymptomatic in most cases.

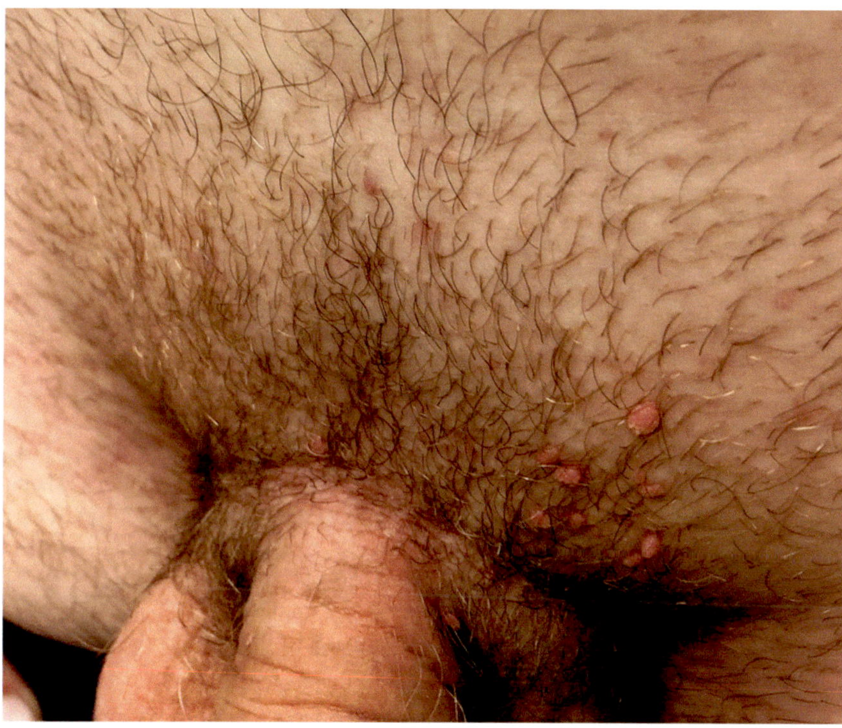

Fig. 13.6 Warts

13.8.1 Management

– Specific treatment includes topical imiquimod 5% cream, 3 times per week for about 16 weeks, podophyllotoxin (0.5% solution) for 3 days on and 4 days off for 6 weeks or sinecatechins (15% ointment) applied three times a day for a maximum of 16 weeks. Cryotherapy can also be used.

13.9 Herpes

– Presents as multiple blisters or erosions. Patient complaints of having burning sensation or pain. Associated with remissions and outbreaks.

– Please see Chap. 6, 'Common Cutaneous Infections' for more details on clinical presentation, diagnosis and management of genital herpes.

13.10 Syphilis

– Caused by *Treponema pallidum*.

– Classically manifests as solitary, painless, indurated ulcer (Chancer). It has an incubation period of 9–90 days.

13.10.1 Diagnosis

– Direct detection of *T. pallidum*, provides definitive evidence of infection. Dark field microscopy, the traditional way of diagnosis has practical limitations. Therefore, direct fluorescence antibody test and polymerase chain reaction (PCR) are the ones that are used for definitive evidence.

– Serology is an indirect method of diagnosing for syphilis. It may be negative in about 30% of primary syphilitic patients (Huber et al. 1983).

– Serologic tests for syphilis comprises of both treponemal tests and nontreponemal tests. Both types of tests are required for an accurate serologic diagnosis of syphilis.

– Treponemal tests detect antibodies to *T. pallidum* itself and these antibodies may be detectable only after 2–4 weeks of exposure (Soreng et al. 2014; Forrestel et al. 2020).

- Results are reported as reactive or nonreactive without any titers.

- While treponemal tests detect antibodies to *T. pallidum* itself, nontreponemal tests detect IgM and IgG antibodies to lipoidal antigens released from damaged host cells and *T. pallidum* (Satyaputra et al. 2021).

- For diagnosis of syphilis, the nontreponemal test is usually performed first. If this is positive, it is followed by a treponemal test for confirmation.

- Venereal Disease Research Laboratory (VDRL) and Rapid Plasma Reagin (RPR) tests are the two most commonly used nontreponemal tests. Both these tests are helpful to diagnose syphilis, and also to monitor response to treatment. These are reported as titers. It takes about 4–5 weeks after infections occurred for them to become reactive (Tuddenham and Zenilman 2019).

- Fluorescent treponemal antibody absorption assay (FTA-ABS), *T. pallidum* hemagglutination test (TPHA), and various treponemal enzyme immunoassays (EIAs) are some of the treponemal tests used.

- If a reactive nontreponemal test result is followed by a reactive treponemal test that confirms the diagnosis of syphilis.

13.10.2 Management

- In adult patients with primary syphilis, benzathine penicillin 2.4 million units administered intra muscularly as single dose is the treatment of choice (P&S Syphilis 2021).

- Doxycycline 100 mg orally twice daily for 14 days or tetracycline 500 mg orally 4 times daily for 14 days can be effective and used if patient is allergic to penicillin and not pregnant. If pregnant, desensitize and administer benzathine penicillin. On the day of treatment, prior to initiating treatment, non treponemal titers need to be obtained. Failure of nontreponemal test titers to reduce by fourfold within 12 months after therapy may be indicative of treatment failure. Therefore, serologic evaluation should be performed at 6 and 12 months after treatment (P&S Syphilis 2021).

13.11 Erythroplasia of Queyrat

- Erythroplasia of Queyrat (EQ) that manifests clinically as a well-defined erythematous plaque on the glans penis is classified as squmous cell carcinoma in situ (Iafrate et al. 2020).

- It is associated with HPV 16 and 8 (Heppt et al. 2019).

- Common in uncircumscribed older males. Clinically it can be confused with simple balanitis. Therefore, lesions that look like balanitis and do not respond to topical steroids should raise the suspicion for EQ. Confirmation is through biopsy.

13.11.1 Management

- Includes topical imiquimod cream, 5-flourauracil cream, cryotherapy. Surgical therapy include local excision (Iafrate et al. 2020).

- Often a referral to dermatologist or urologist is warranted upon suspicion of this condition.

Bibliography

Blaise G, Nikkels AF, Hermanns-Lê T, Nikkels-Tassoudji N, Piérard GE. Corynebacterium-associated skin infections. Int J Dermatol. 2008;47(9):884–90.

Craddock LN, Schieke SM. Superficial Fungal Infection. In: Kang S, Amagai M, Bruckner AL, Enk AH, Margolis DJ, McMichael AJ, Orringer JS, editors. Fitzpatrick's dermatology, vol. 9e. New York, NY: McGraw-Hill Education; 2019.

Forrestel AK, Kovarik CL, Katz KA. Sexually acquired syphilis: laboratory diagnosis, management, and prevention. J Am Acad Dermatol. 2020;82(1):17–28.

Gudjonsson JE, Elder JT. Psoriasis. In: Kang S, Amagai M, Bruckner AL, Enk AH, Margolis DJ, McMichael AJ, Orringer JS, editors. Fitzpatrick's dermatology, vol. 9e. New York, NY: McGraw-Hill Education; 2019.

Heppt MV, Schlager G, Berking C. Epithelial precancerous lesions. In: Kang S, Amagai M, Bruckner AL, Enk AH, Margolis DJ, McMichael AJ, Orringer JS, editors. Fitzpatrick's dermatology, 9e. New York, NY: McGraw-Hill Education; 2019.

Holdiness MR. Management of cutaneous erythrasma. Drugs. 2002;62(8):1131–41.

Honigman AD, Dubin DP, Chu J, Lin MJ. Management of pearly penile papules: a review of the literature. J Cutan Med Surg. 2019;24(1):79–85.

Huber TW, Storms S, Pl Y, Phillips L, Rogers TE, Moore DG, et al. Reactivity of microhemagglutination, fluorescent treponemal antibody absorption, Venereal Disease Research Laboratory, and rapid plasma reagin tests in primary syphilis. J Clin Microbiol. 1983;17(3):405–9.

Iafrate M, Mancini M, Prayer Galetti T, Szekely S, Zattra E, Vaccari D et al. Efficacy of topical photodynamic therapy in the treatment of erythroplasia of Queyrat. Dermatol Rep. 2020;12(1).

Kirtschig G. Lichen sclerosus—presentation, diagnosis and management. Deutsches Aerzteblatt Online. 2016

O'Gorman SM, Torgerson RR. Allergic contact dermatitis of the vulva. Dermatitis. 2013;24(2):64–72.

P&S Syphilis. STI Treatment Guidelines. www.cdc.gov (2021). https://www.cdc.gov/std/treatment-guidelines/p-and-s-syphilis.htm. Accessed 20 Oct 2021

Satyaputra F, Hendry S, Braddick M, Sivabalan P, Norton R. The laboratory diagnosis of syphilis. J Clin Microbiol. 2021;59(10):1128.

Shumway NK. Skin diseases of the genitals and perineum. In: Soutor C, Hordinsky MK, editors. Clinical dermatology: diagnosis and management of common disorders, vol. 2e. New York, NY: McGraw-Hill Education; 2022.

Soreng K, Levy R, Fakile Y. Serologic testing for syphilis: benefits and challenges of a reverse algorithm. Clin Microbiol Newsl. 2014;36(24):195–202.

Taudorf EH, Jemec GBE, Hay RJ, Saunte DML. Cutaneous candidiasis—an evidence-based review of topical and systemic treatments to inform clinical practice. J Eur Acad Dermatol Venereol JEADV. 2019;3(10):1863–73.

Tuddenham SA, Zenilman JM. Syphilis. In: Kang S, Amagai M, Bruckner AL, Enk AH, Margolis DJ, McMichael AJ, Orringer JS, editors. Fitzpatrick's dermatology, vol. 9e. New York, NY: McGraw-Hill Education; 2019.

van de kerkhof PCM, Murphy GM, Austad J, Ljungberg A, Cambazard F, BouératDuvold L. Psoriasis of the face and flexures. J Dermatol Treatm. 2007;18(6):351–60.

Chapter 14
Legs

Abstract This chapter provides an overview of the common dermatological conditions, such as cutaneous small vessel vasculitis, asteatotic eczema erythema nodosum, that can occur on the legs. The chapter discusses mainly from their clinical perspective. It provides details about the clinical presentation of these conditions and ways to diagnose them; where appropriate, it provides clinical information regarding how to diagnose them clinically. It also discusses their treatment options and the circumstances as to when the patients need to be referred to the dermatologist.

Keywords Vasculitis · Erythema nodosum · Asteatotic eczema · Stasis dermatitis · Lichen simplex chronicus · Atopic dermatitis

14.1 Cutaneous Small Vessel Vasculitis (CSVV)

- Cutaneous vasculitis (Fig. 14.1) that involves small-sized vessels and is limited to the skin is often described as CSVV (Jennette et al. 2012; Goeser et al. 2014).

- Clinically it manifests classically as palpable purpura. Other lesions such as petechiae, urticarial papules, hemorrhagic vesicles and pustules can also be seen (Micheletti 2022).

- Most commonly lower extremities are involved. Area of trauma or pressure can also be affected.

- The etiology is idiopathic in 50% of the cases.

- Drugs such as β-lactams and other antibiotics, upper respiratory infections, Group A streptococcus and hepatitis C are among those infections that can trigger (Micheletti and Werth 2015).

D. K. Yellumahanthi, *Manual of Primary Care Dermatology*,
https://doi.org/10.1007/978-3-031-68406-7_14

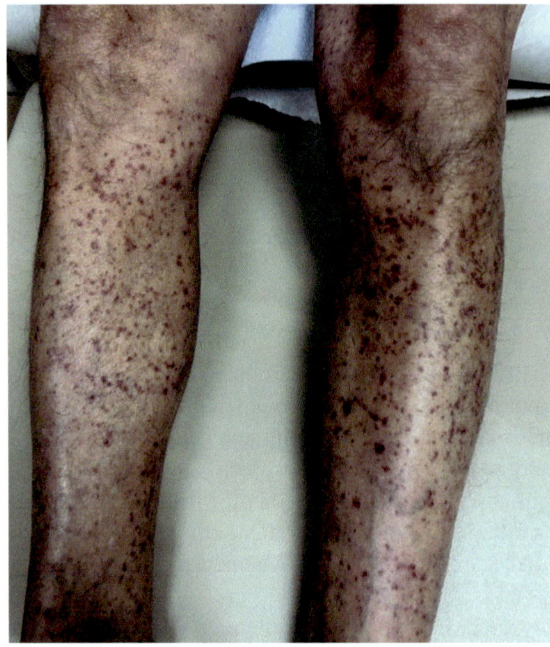

Fig. 14.1 Cutaneous small vessel vasculitis

- **Diagnosis:** When typical purpuric lesions are present in lower extremities, the diagnosis is obvious clinically. Histopathology can help in diagnosing CSVV, in scenarios where clinical presentation is ambiguous.

14.1.1 Management

- It is usually self-limited. About 10% of cases can become chronic or recurrent (Russell and Gibson 2006).

- Aggressive treatment is usually not needed. Eliminating any triggers need to be done. Topical moderate-to-potent steroids for itching can be prescribed. Oral prednisone can be administered in cases that have extensive involvement.

14.2 Stasis Dermatitis (Fig. 14.2)

- Caused by chronic venous insufficiency.

- It presents with bilateral erythematous, eczematous plaques usually involving the lower one third of the leg, more so around the medial malleolus (Zepecki and Blasiak 2018).

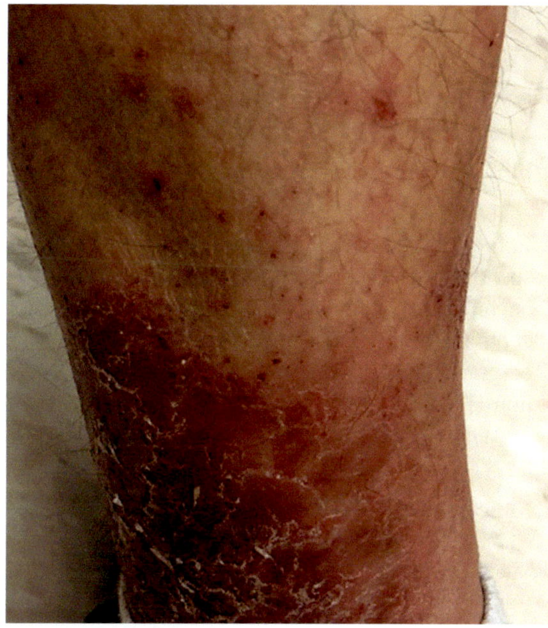

Fig. 14.2 Stasis dermatitis

- Usually associated with edema of the lower legs.

14.2.1 Management

- Includes elevation of the leg and compression stockings.
- Unna boot, a bandage that contains moist zinc oxide, was found to be beneficial. It improves the pruritus, inflammation and eczema. It can also be combined with topical corticosteroids (Yosipovitch et al. 2023).
- Mid-potency topical steroids or high potent topical corticosteroids can be used (Yosipovitch et al. 2023).
- Usage of emollients also needs to be encouraged.
- Referral to vascular surgeon to address the underlying venous insufficiency is a vital component of management (Sundaresan et al. 2017).

14.3 Erythema Nodosum (EN) (Fig. 14.3)

- EN is a type of panniculitis.

- Etiology is precisely unknown.

- In most cases, EN is primary or idiopathic. However, it can be due to infections such as tuberculosis, streptococcal infections, infectious mononucleosis, herpes, hepatitis B, systemic fungal infections or drugs such as sulfonamides, oral contraceptives, penicillin, minocycline, salicylates or inflammatory bowel diseases or granulomatous diseases like sarcoidosis. Malignancies such as Hodgkin's, non-Hodgkin's lymphoma and leukemia can also cause EN (Pérez-Garza et al. 2021).

- More common in females.

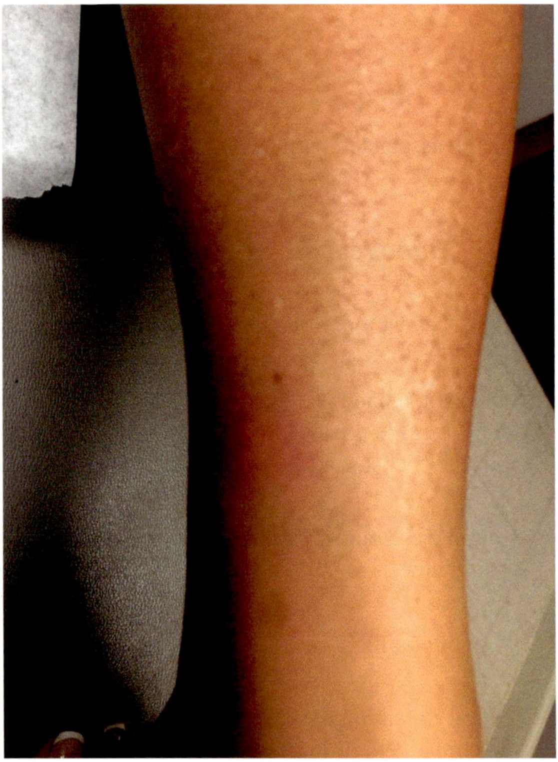

Fig. 14.3 Erythema nodosum

14.3.1 Clinical Features

- Characterized by the appearance of painful or tender erythematous nodules on the lower legs, commonly.
- Usually bilateral and symmetric.
- Lesions could turn different colors such as violaceous, brown, green or yellow as they age and resemble bruises.
- Often systemic symptoms such as fever, arthralgia, headache and gastrointestinal symptoms can be present (Pérez-Garza et al. 2021).
- Course of the EN depends on etiology. Lesions are usually self-limiting. May last for about 1–6 weeks. Please keep in mind, new lesions could occur during this time. Therefore, patient needs to be informed about it.
- Lesions do not ulcerate and heal without scarring.

14.3.2 Management

- Bed rest, compression stockings, anti-inflammatory drugs can be used for symptomatic relief. In secondary EN cases, the cause needs to be treated. Similarly, any offending drugs to be stopped.

14.4 Lichen Simplex Chronicus (LSC) (Fig. 14.4)

- It can be classified as a type of endogenous eczema.
- Usually manifests as an itchy, isolated, circumscribed, lichenified plaque.
- Repetitive rubbing and scratching is often a triggering factor.
- Common areas are nape of the neck, scalp, ankles, lower part of the legs (ankles, lateral part of the shin), upper thighs, outer aspects of the forearms and wrists, vulva, pubis, anal area, scrotum (Lichen Simplex 2022).

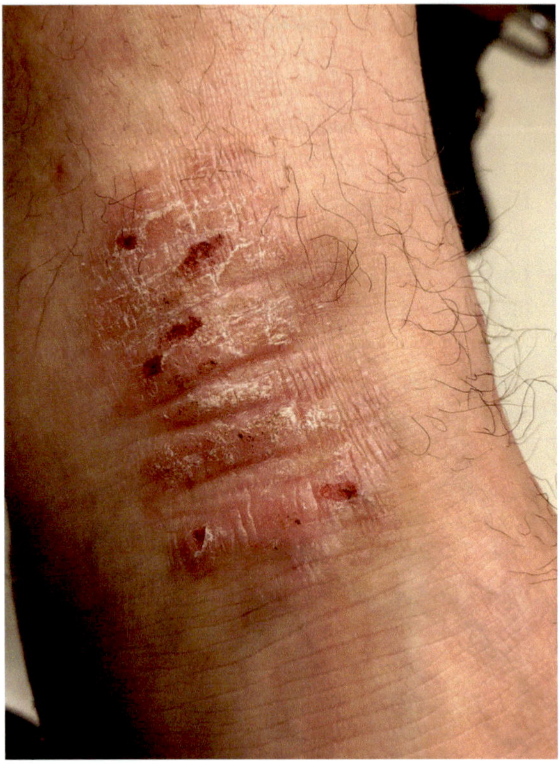

Fig. 14.4 Lichen simplex chronicus

14.4.1 Management

- Foremost important aspect of management is educating the patient about stopping the rubbing and scratching. Topical potent steroids with or without occlusion are helpful.

- Intralesional triamcinolone can also be used in cases not responding to the above measures (Lichen Simplex 2022).

14.5 Nummular Eczema (Nummular Dermatitis) (Discoid Eczema)

- Usually manifests on extremities, as erythematous plaques that are coin shaped (Fig. 14.5).

- Bilaterally symmetrical presentation is common.

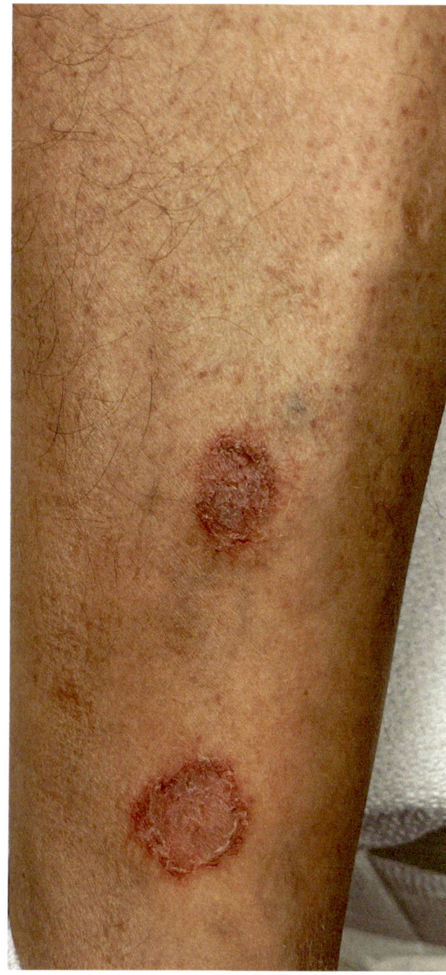

Fig. 14.5 Nummular eczema

- Common in lower extremities followed by upper extremities (Leung et al. 2021).
- Relapses are common.

14.5.1 Management

- Topical potent corticosteroids and super potent steroids also can be used (Leung et al. 2021).
- Emollient usage also needs to be encouraged.

14.6 Asteatotic Eczema (Eczema Craquele)

- It is a type of endogenous eczema.
- It is characterized by itchy, dry, fissured skin with scales (Fig. 14.6).
- The fissured skin manifests in a curvilinear pattern.
- There is usually underlying xerosis.
- Anterolateral aspects of the lower legs are a common site. Arms and back of the trunk are the other common sites (Specht and Persaud 2023).
- Typically presents in the elderly during the winter seasons.

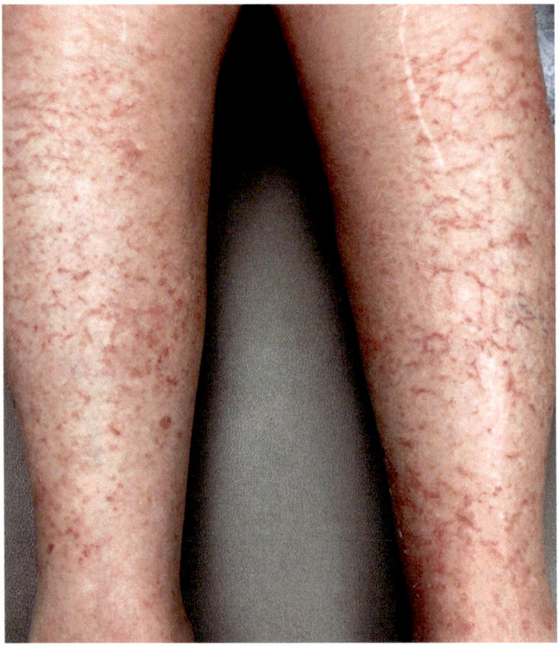

Fig. 14.6 Asteatotic eczema

14.6.1 Management

- Includes application of daily emollients. Antihistamines and topical corticosteroids can be used.

14.7 Atopic Dermatitis (AD) (Fig. 14.7)

Please see Chap. 5, 'Eczema', for more details on its clinical presentation and management.

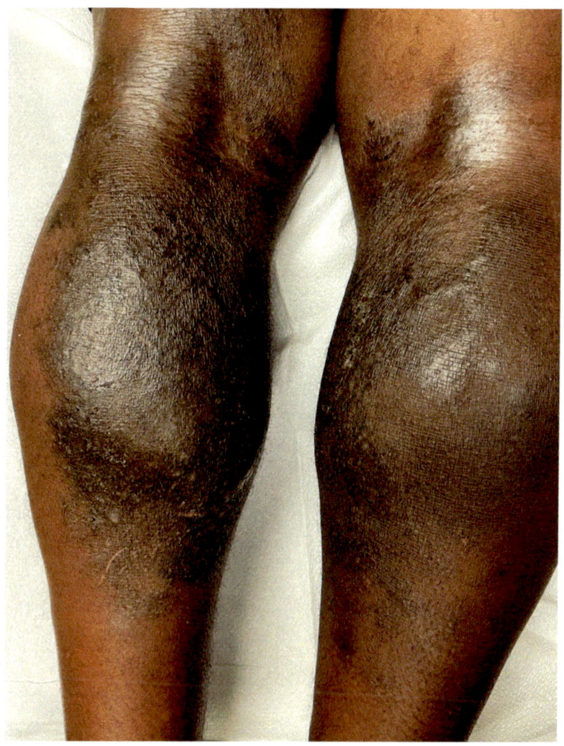

Fig. 14.7 Atopic dermatitis in adult

14.8 Psoriasis Vulgaris (Fig. 14.8)

Psoriasis vulgaris is a common papulosquamous disorder (scaly dermatosis). Its distribution and appearance are quite distinct. A common form of it, psoriasis vulgaris, can occur on the shins. Examining other common areas where it can occur (such as back of elbows, lumbosacral area) can help in its clinical diagnosis.

Please see Chap. 3, 'Papulosquamous Disorders', for more details on its clinical presentation and management.

Please note that any infections discussed in Chap. 6, 'Common Cutaneous Infections', can also occur on legs.

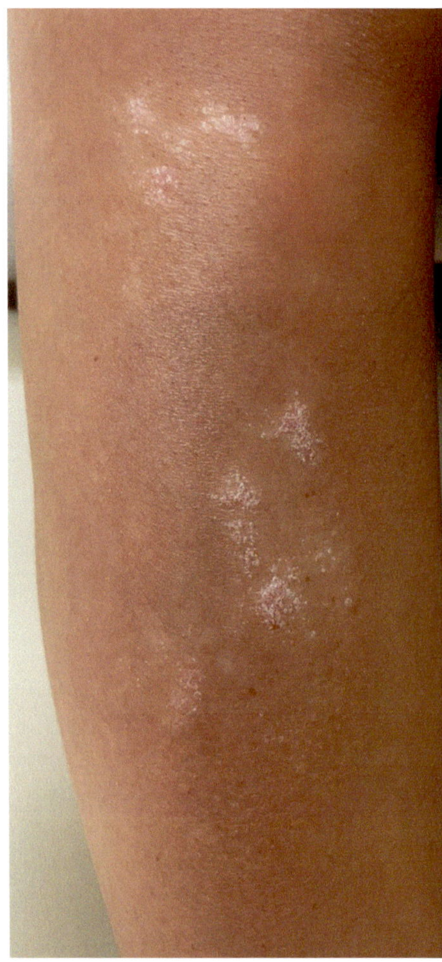

Fig. 14.8 Psoriasis vulgaris

Bibliography

Goeser MR, Laniosz V, Wetter DA. A practical approach to the diagnosis, evaluation, and management of cutaneous small-vessel vasculitis. Am J Clin Dermatol. 2014;15(4):299–306.

Jennette JC, Falk RJ, Bacon PA, Basu N, Cid MC, Ferrario F, et al. Revised International Chapel Hill consensus conference nomenclature of vasculitides. Arthritis Rheum. 2012;65(1):1–11.

Leung AKC, Lam JM, Leong KF, Leung AAM, Wong AHC, Hon KL. Nummular eczema: an updated review. Recent Pat Inflam Allergy Drug Discov. 2021;14(2):146–55.

Lichen Simplex. DermNet NZ. dermnetnz.org; 2022. https://dermnetnz.org/topics/lichen-simplex

Micheletti RG. Cutaneous small vessel vasculitis: a practical guide to diagnosis and management. Am J Clin Dermatol. 2022;24(1):89.

Micheletti RG, Werth VP. Small vessel vasculitis of the skin. Rheum Dis Clin North America. 2015;41(1):21–32.

Pérez-Garza DM, Chavez-Alvarez S, Ocampo-Candiani J, Gomez-Flores M. Erythema nodosum: a practical approach and diagnostic algorithm. Am J Clin Dermatol. 2021;22(3):367–78.

Russell JP, Gibson LE. Primary cutaneous small vessel vasculitis: approach to diagnosis and treatment. Int J Dermatol. 2006;45(1):3–13.

Specht S, Persaud Y (2023) Asteatotic eczema. In: StatPearls. StatPearls Publishing, Treasure Island (FL) (2024). PMID: 31747214

Sundaresan S, Migden MR, Silapunt S. Stasis dermatitis: pathophysiology, evaluation, and management. Am J Clin Dermatol. 2017;18(3):383–90.

Yosipovitch G, Nedorost ST, Silverberg JI, Friedman AJ, Canosa JM, Cha A. Stasis dermatitis: an overview of its clinical presentation, pathogenesis, and management. Am J Clin Dermatol. 2023;24(2):275–86.

Zepecki AK, Blasiak R. Stasis dermatitis: differentiation from other common causes of lower leg inflammation and management strategies. Curr Geriatr Rep. 2018;7(4):222–7.

Chapter 15
Feet

Abstract This chapter provides an overview of the common dermatological conditions such as tinea pedis, psoriasis and contact dermatitis that can occur on the feet. The chapter discusses mainly from their clinical perspective. It provides details about the clinical presentation of these conditions and ways to diagnose them; where feasible, it provides clinical information regarding how to diagnose them clinically. It also discusses their treatment options and when appropriate the circumstances as to when the patients need to be referred to the dermatologist.

Keywords Tinea pedis · Athlete's foot · Psoriasis · Callosity and corns · Warts · Erythrasma · Candidal intertrigo · Pompholyx

15.1 Tinea Pedis (Athlete's Foot)

– Dermatophytic infection of the feet.

15.1.1 Clinical Manifestations

– Can manifest as either interdigital or chronic hyperkeratotic (moccasin) or bullous (vesicular) or ulcerative form (Ilkit and Durdu 2014).

– Interdigital form is the most common form. It presents with scaling, erythema, maceration affecting the lateral toe clefts.

– Moccasin type (Fig. 15.1) presents as diffuse or focal scaling on the soles and the medial and lateral aspects of the feet, in a distribution similar to a moccasin footwear. The erythema is usually mild but is variable (Craddock and Schieke 2019).

– The vesicular form (Fig. 15.2) manifests as vesicles or pustules or bullae commonly involving either mid anterior plantar surface or near the instep.

D. K. Yellumahanthi, *Manual of Primary Care Dermatology*,
https://doi.org/10.1007/978-3-031-68406-7_15

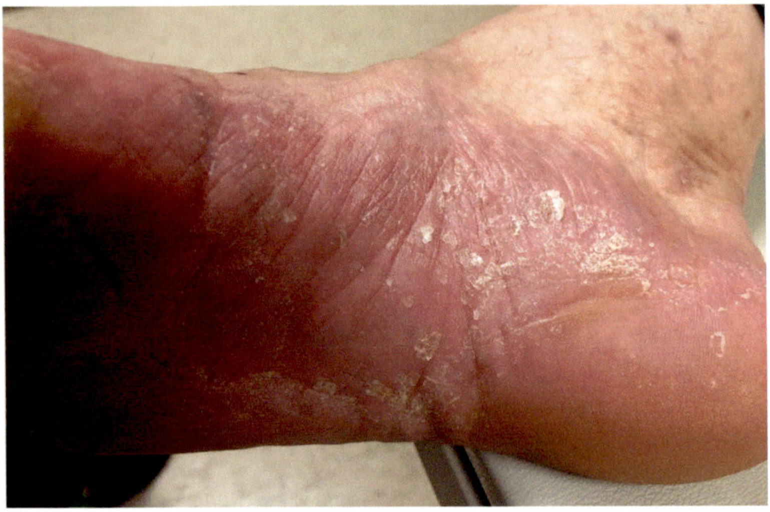

Fig. 15.1 Tinea pedis (moccasin distribution)

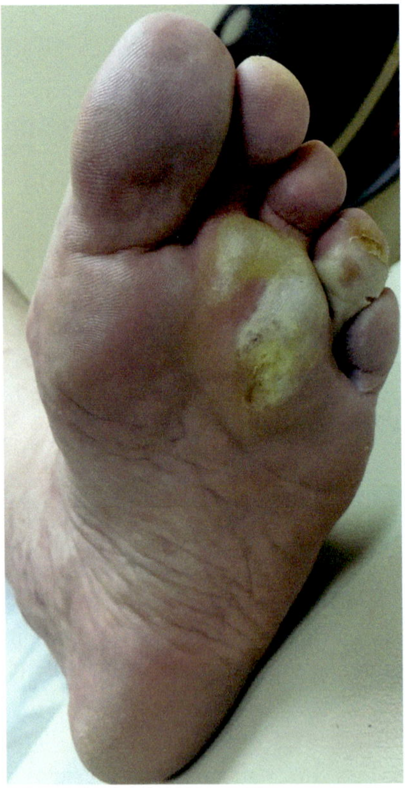

Fig. 15.2 Tinea pedis, blister form

– The ulcerative type is an exacerbation of the interdigital form. It is most often seen in diabetics or immunocompromised individuals (Legge et al. 2008).

15.1.2 Diagnosis

– A potassium hydroxide (KOH) prep can be performed in the office to confirm the diagnosis.

– A culture for fungus can also be done.

– A skin biopsy can also be done to confirm the diagnosis.

15.1.3 Management

– Topical antifungal therapy is the mainstay of treatment for superficial or localized tinea pedis (Leung et al. 2023).

– Topical clotrimazole, miconazole, ketoconazole, oxiconazole, sulconazole, sertaconazole, luliconazole, terbinafine and ciclopirox are the options.

– Oral treatment can be considered if topical antifungal treatment is not effective or if the condition is extensive or in immunocompromised patients or if onychomycosis coexists (Rajagopalan et al. 2018).

– Oral terbinafine daily (250 mg for adults) for two weeks and fluconazole 150 mg po q weekly for 2–6 weeks are among the regimens used (Mahajan and Sahoo 2016).

– Supportive measures such as limiting the use of occluded footwear need to be discussed.

15.2 Psoriasis

– Palms and plantar surface (Fig. 15.3) can be involved with psoriasis as a part of chronic plaque type of psoriasis or as a separate entity, palmoplantar psoriasis (PP). PP can manifest as psoriasis localized to the palms and soles; it can occur in various forms ranging from predominant pustular form to hyperkeratotic scaly plaques (Engin et al. 2017; Farley et al. 2009; Menter and Griffiths 2007).

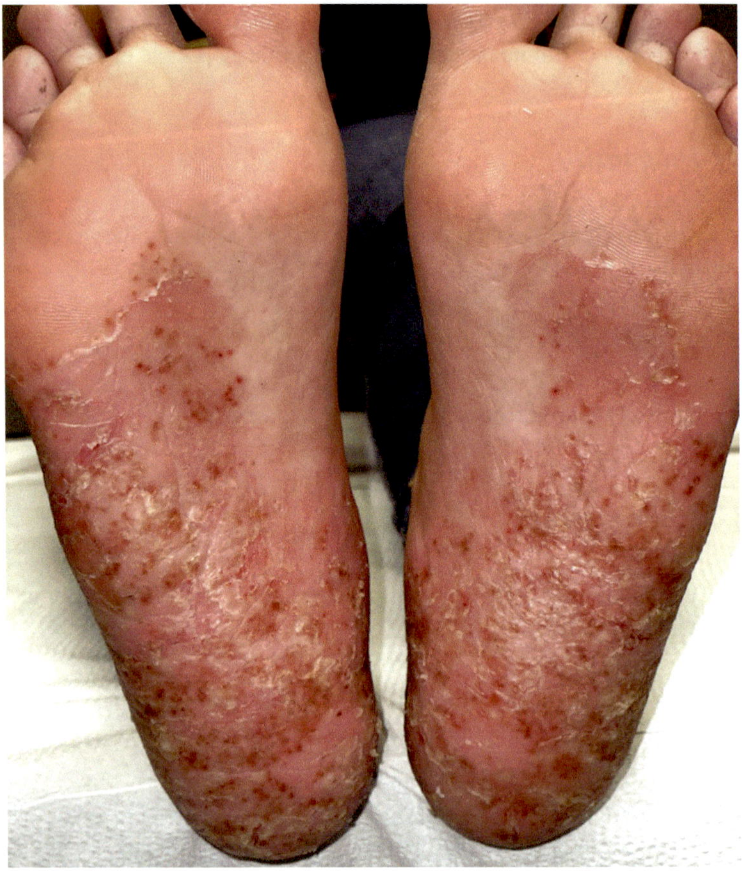

Fig. 15.3 Plantar psoriasis: erythematous plaques with minute superficial pustules

15.2.1 Diagnosis

- Differentiation from tinea pedis (T. pedis): Psoriasis of feet is easy to differentiate from tinea pedis if other classical sites such as back of elbows, front of knees, lumbosacral region are involved. If not, sometimes diagnosis can be challenging.
- Even if all other classical areas are not involved, usually palms are involved with plantar psoriasis as a part of palmoplantar psoriasis. Therefore, examination of the palms needs to be done.
- Nail changes such as subungual hyperkeratosis and onycholysis can be present in both T. pedis and psoriasis. Nail pitting could favor the diagnosis toward psoriasis.

- KOH prep or culture for fungus can rule in or rule out T. pedis.

- Skin biopsy can confirm psoriasis.

15.2.2 Management

- Topical ultra(super)potent steroids such as clobetasol ointment are often first line of drugs used. Calcipotriene or calcineurin inhibitors can also be used as steroid sparing agents. The combination of corticosteroids with calcipotriol is found to be more effective than monotherapy (Handa 2010).

- If topical therapy is not effective, phototherapy, systemic retinoids and biological drugs can be used. Often it is best to refer to dermatology if not effective with topical medications.

- Please see Chap. 3, 'Papulosquamous Disorders', for more details on its clinical presentation and management.

15.3 Contact Dermatitis

- Involves the dorsal area of the feet more than the plantar side.

- Can manifest as either erythematous patches or blisters (in acute cases).

- If contact dermatitis is suspected, allergic dermatitis to footwear needs to be ruled out, first.

15.3.1 Management

- Avoidance of potential allergen is a key component of management. Topical potent steroids such as betamethasone dipropionate 0.05% ointment can be used to treat the skin lesions.

15.4 Corns (Fig. 15.4)

- It is cone-shaped with circumscribed hyperkeratosis of the skin over the bony prominence. Its apex is pointed inward and presses on the surrounding structures. It can cause pain while walking due to pressure on the nearby nerves. For the same reason, applying pressure vertically can elicit pain, a sign often aids in the diagnosis of corn (Farndon et al. 2013).

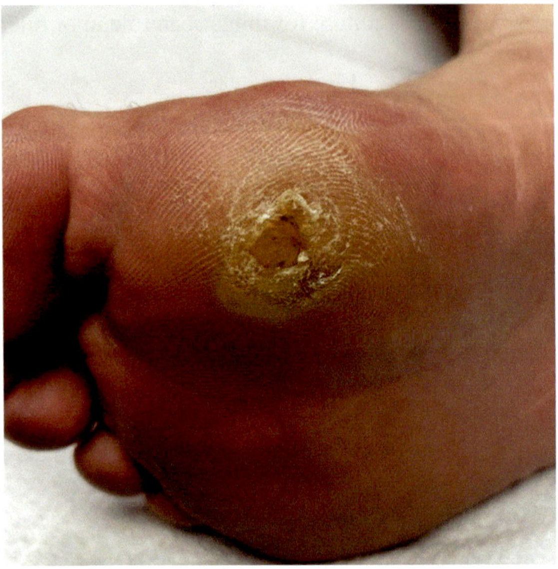

Fig. 15.4 Corn

15.4.1 Diagnosis

- Diagnosis is made clinically. Paring of the surface can make the underlying central white core of the corn visible.

- The fact that they are painful, the presence of central white core of corn and absence of black dots (thrombosed capillaries) should help in differentiating from warts.

15.4.2 Management

- Avoidance of ill-fitting shoes to relieve pressure on it is recommended. Gentle paring of the lesion can help. Topical 40% salicylic acid plasters can be used (Farndon et al. 2013).

- If not responding to conservative measures, a referral to podiatrist may be needed to explore for any surgical intervention.

15.5 Callosity (Fig. 15.5)

- It is formed as a result of repeated pressure or friction at a particular site.

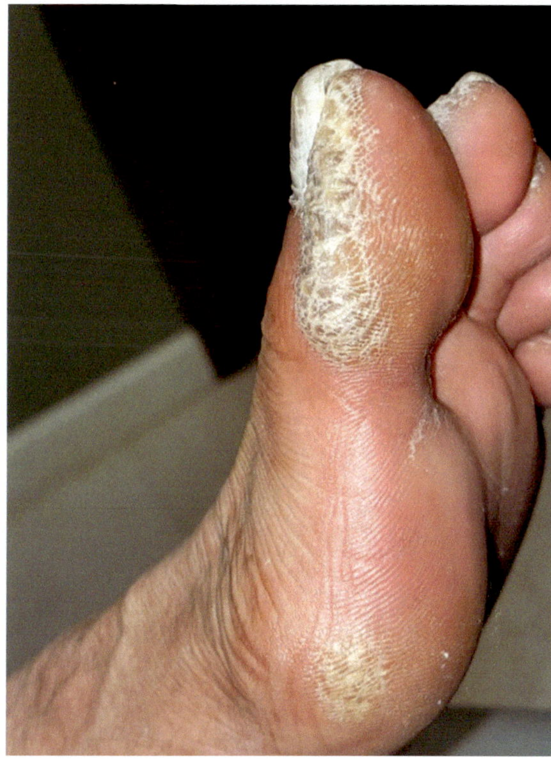

Fig. 15.5 Callosity

– It is manifested as an area of circumscribed hyperkeratosis of the skin. The thickest part is usually in the center. It gradually tapers off to the periphery merging to the surrounding normal skin (Mehtha et al. 2013).

15.5.1 Diagnosis

– Diagnosis is made clinically. Unlike corn, it is not painful and is devoid of the central white core. It can be differentiated from warts by the fact that they do not disrupt the normal skin lines and are devoid of the black dots (thrombosed capillaries) on its surface.

15.5.2 Management

– It includes making sure that the repeated friction is minimized or stopped. Topical application of urea paste and salicylic acid can help.

15.6 Plantar Warts (Fig. 15.6)

Warts can also occur near nail folds—periungual warts (Fig. 15.7).

- Please see Chap. 6, 'Common Cutaneous Infections', for details on its clinical presentation and management.

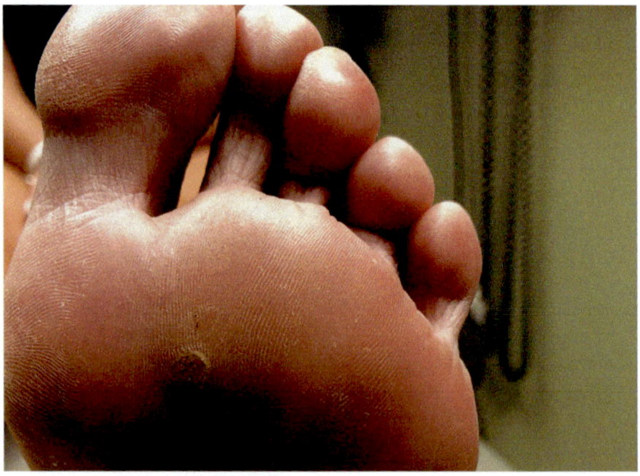

Fig. 15.6 Plantar wart

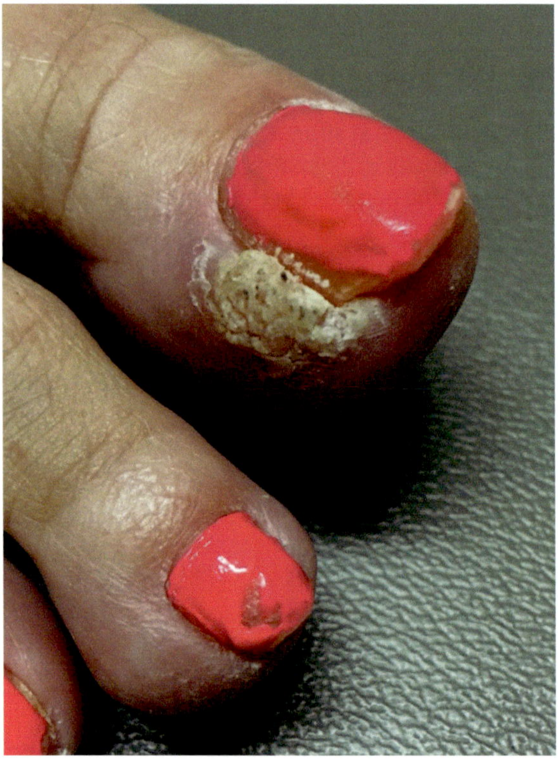

Fig. 15.7 Periungual wart

15.7 Pompholyx (Dyshidrotic Eczema)

- Manifests as vesicles only on the sides of the fingers or toes.

- It can be associated with recurrences.

15.7.1 Management

- It includes usage of super potent topical corticosteroids like clobetasol propionate 0.05% ointment.

- Please see Chap. 11, 'Upper Extremity Including Hands', Fig. 15.9 for a picture of pompholyx and Chap. 5, 'Eczema', for more details on its clinical presentation, diagnosis and management.

15.8 Erythrasma

- Please see Chap. 6, 'Common Cutaneous Infections', for details on its clinical presentation, diagnosis and management.

15.9 Candidal Intertrigo (Fig. 15.8)

- Please see Chap. 6, 'Common Cutaneous Infections', for more details on its clinical presentation and management.

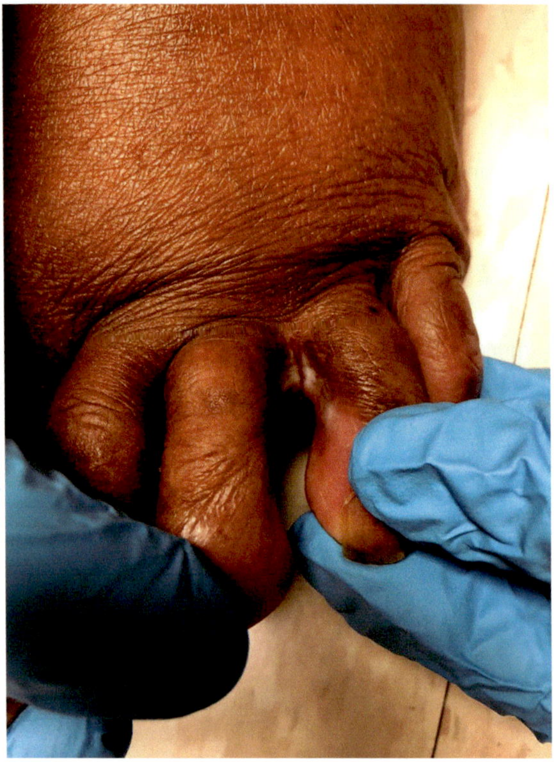

Fig. 15.8 Candidal intertrigo

15.10 Cutaneous Small Vessel Vasculitis (CSVV) (Fig. 15.9)

- Please see Chap. 14, 'Legs', for details on its clinical presentation, diagnosis and management.

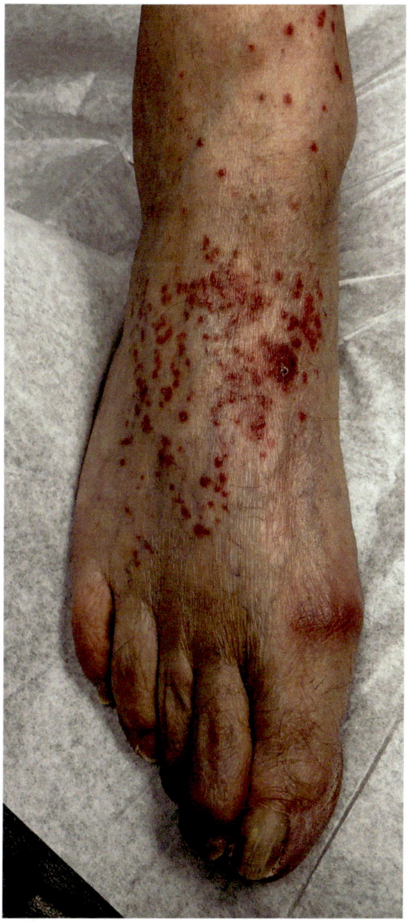

Fig. 15.9 Cutaneous small vessel vasculitis

Bibliography

Craddock LN, Schieke SM. Superficial fungal infection. In: Kang S, Amagai M, Bruckner AL, Enk AH, Margolis DJ, McMichael AJ, Orringer JS, editors. Fitzpatrick's dermatology, 9e. New York, NY: McGraw-Hill Education; 2019.
Engin B, Aşkın Ö, Tüzün Y. Palmoplantar psoriasis. Clin Dermatol. 2017;35(1):19–27.
Farley E, Masrour Shamin, McKey J, Menter A. Palmoplantar psoriasis: a phenotypical and clinical review with introduction of a new quality-of-life assessment tool. J Am Acad Dermatol. 2009;60(6):1024–31.
Farndon LJ, Vernon W, Walters SJ, Dixon S, Bradburn M, Concannon M, et al. The effectiveness of salicylic acid plasters compared with "usual" scalpel debridement of corns: a randomised controlled trial. J Foot Ankle Res. 2013;6(1):1–8.
Handa S. Newer trends in the management of psoriasis at difficult to treat locations: Scalp, palmoplantar disease and nails. Indian J Dermatol Venereol Leprol. 2010;76(6):634.
Ilkit M, Durdu M. Tinea pedis: The etiology and global epidemiology of a common fungal infection. Crit Rev Microbiol. 2014;41(3):374–88.

Legge BS, Grady JF, Lacey AM. The incidence of Tinea Pedis in diabetic versus nondiabetic patients with interdigital macerations. J Am Podiatr Med Assoc. 2008;98(5):353–6.
Leung AK, Barankin B, Lam JM, Leong KF, Hon KL. Tinea pedis: an updated review. Drugs Context. 2023;12:2023–51.
Mahajan R, Sahoo A. Management of tinea corporis, tinea cruris, and tinea pedis: a comprehensive review. Indian Dermatol Online J. 2016;7(2):77.
Mehtha T, Neela V, Bhuptani SP. Disorders of keratinization. In: Sacchidanand S, Oberoi C, Inamadar A, editors. IADVL textbook of dermatology. 4th ed. New York, NY: Wiley; 2013.
Menter A, Griffiths CE. Current and future management of psoriasis. Lancet (London, England). 2007;370(9583):272–84.
Rajagopalan M, Inamadar A, Mittal A, Miskeen AK, Srinivas CR, Sardana K, et al. Expert consensus on the management of dermatophytosis in India (ECTODERM India). BMC Dermatol. 2018;18(1):1–11.

Chapter 16
Common Disorders of Nails

Abstract This chapter provides an overview of the common nail disorders such as onychomycosis that are commonly encountered by primary care providers. The chapter discusses mainly from their clinical perspective. It provides details about the clinical presentation of these conditions and ways to diagnose them; where feasible, it provides clinical information regarding how to diagnose them clinically. It also discusses their treatment options and where appropriate the circumstances as to when the patients need to be referred to the dermatologist. The chapter also provides signs that are commonly associated with nail melanoma.

Keywords Subungual hyperkeratosis · Onycholysis · Nail pitting · Onychomycosis · Nail psoriasis · Acute and chronic paronychia · Subungual hematoma · Longitudinal melanocytic nevus · Nail melanoma

This chapter provides an overview of the following conditions that affect the nail apparatus:

Subungual hyperkeratosis.
Onycholysis.
Nail pitting.
Onychomycosis.
Psoriasis.
Pseudomonas.
Acute and chronic paronychia.
Subungual hematoma.
Longitudinal melanocytic nevus.
Nail melanoma.

16.1 Anatomy of the Nail Apparatus

- The nail apparatus consists of the nail plate, nail matrix, nail bed, the proximal and lateral nail folds and the hyponychium.

D. K. Yellumahanthi, *Manual of Primary Care Dermatology*,
https://doi.org/10.1007/978-3-031-68406-7_16

Nail plate: The nail plate is a hard structure that acts as a protective covering by preventing trauma to the tips of toes and fingers.

Nail bed lies beneath the nail plate.

Nail matrix: Most of the nail matrix lies beneath the proximal nail fold. The distal third of the nail matrix can be visible through the proximal portion of the nail plate as lunula, a half-moon-shaped structure.

Hyponychium: It is located at the distal free edge of the nail plate just proximal to the distal groove. It is contiguous with the volar skin.

16.2 Subungual Hyperkeratosis

Hyperkeratosis of the nail bed (Fig. 16.1) is a frequent event. It is characteristic for onychomycosis and psoriasis. Other frequent causes are trauma, allergic, toxic contact and atopic dermatitis. It is usually always associated with onycholysis which is separation of nail plate from distal nail bed (Hanake 2019).

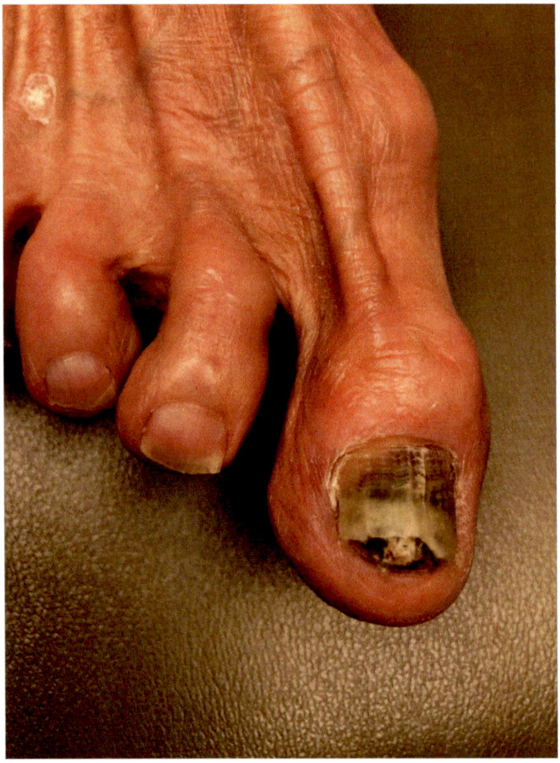

Fig. 16.1 Subungual hyperkeratosis

16.3 Onycholysis

- Detachment of the nail plate from the distal nail bed is called onycholysis.
- All conditions with abnormal subungual hyperkeratosis will eventually lead to onycholysis (Haneke 2019).
- Causes: Onychomycosis and psoriasis are the important ones. Trauma can also cause onycholysis.

16.3.1 Management

- For inflammatory causes such as psoriasis, topical steroid solution or intralesional steroids can be used. If psoriatic onycholysis is refractory to those measures, systemic therapy can be considered. Please see under psoriasis nail in this chapter for more details on management of psoriasis.
- If secondary to onychomycosis, antifungals can be prescribed. Please read onychomycosis in this chapter for more details on management of onychomycosis.
- Traumatic: Trim the nail so that only the adherent part is left and provide supportive therapy until the nail regrows.

16.4 Nail Pitting (Fig. 16.2)

- Depressions in the nail plate with varying distribution and morphology.
- Notable conditions where pitting can be seen are psoriasis, alopecia areata and eczema.

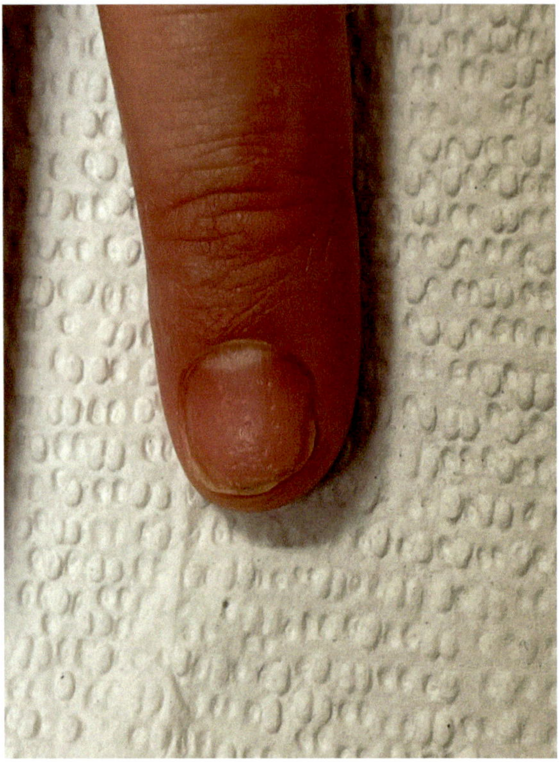

Fig. 16.2 Nail pitting

16.5 Onychomycosis

- Onychomycosis (Fig. 16.3) is the most frequent nail disorder making up approximately 50% of all nail diseases (Gupta et al. 2017).

- Dermatophytes, yeasts and non-dermatophyte molds are the pathogens (Gupta et al. 2017).

Fig. 16.3 Onychomycosis

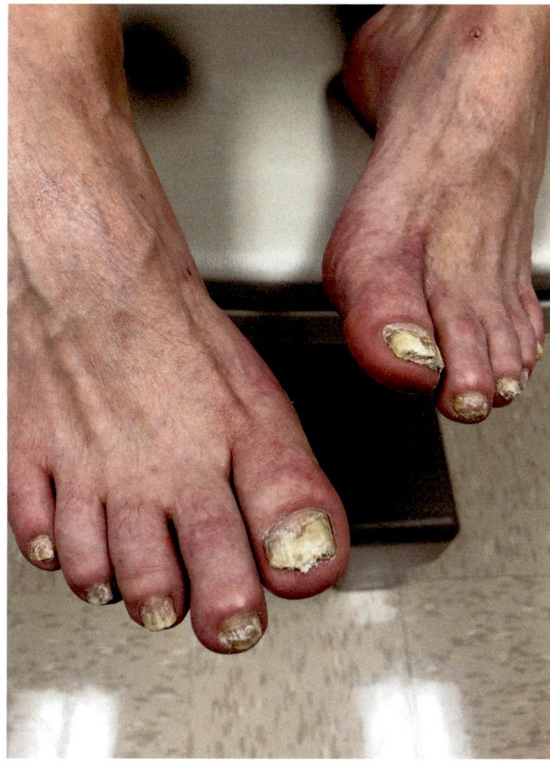

16.5.1 Clinical Features

- Onychomycosis can manifest as various forms. Mainly four types of onychomycosis are recognized based on the clinical presentation and the route of invasion: Distal-lateral subungual onychomycosis (DSO), proximal subungual onychomycosis (PSO), white superficial and candida are the four patterns of infection (Elewski 1998).

- DSO is the most common among them. Proximal subungual onychomycosis is more common in HIV and immunocompromised patients (Elewski 1998).

- In general, the nail changes associated with onychomycosis can include subungual hyperkeratosis, onycholysis and discoloration of nail plate. Onychodystrophy can also occur (Elewski 1998).

16.5.2 Diagnosis

- Although most onychomycoses can be diagnosed clinically, confirmation of the diagnosis can be done by potassium hydroxide microscopic examination of the nail scrapings, histopathology, fungal culture, polymerase chain reaction and flow cytometry (Gupta et al. 2017).

- Among these, culture and microscopy are considered as gold standard (Gupta et al. 2017).

- Nail psoriasis is the most important in differential diagnosis. Presence of nail pitting or arthritis or classical psoriatic skin changes tilts the diagnosis in favor of psoriasis. When in doubt, the above-mentioned confirmatory testing can be done.

16.5.3 Management

- It is important to confirm the diagnosis by any of the above-mentioned methods before starting the treatment. After the treatment also, mycological cure needs to be confirmed.

- Oral antifungals are usually needed.

  Terbinafine, itraconazole and fluconazole are the commonly used drugs. Terbinafine adult dose is 250 mg once daily for about 12 weeks for toenail and 6 weeks for finger nails (Preda-Naumescu et al. 2021).

- Itraconazole can be used as continuous or pulse therapy with similar efficacy (Preda-Naumescu et al. 2021) among adults.

  Continuous regimen consists of 200 mg orally once daily for 12 weeks (toe nails) and 6 weeks for finger nail (Preda-Naumescu et al. 2021).

  Pulse therapy for toenails include 200 mg orally twice daily for 1 week and then no treatment for 3 weeks. This is repeated for 3–4 months (Preda-Naumescu et al. 2021).

- Fluconazole 150 mg/week is used off label for onychomycosis.

- When oral treatment cannot be given, the topicals approved to use include 5% tavaborole, 8% ciclopirox lacquer and 10% efinaconazole (Carley et al. 2017).

- Among these, relatively efinaconazole 10% solution is reported to have increased efficacy (Gupta et al. 2017; LaSenna 2015).

16.6 Nail Psoriasis

16.6.1 Clinical Presentation

- Can manifest as subungual hyperkeratosis, onycholysis, pitting.
- Focal onycholysis can sometimes present as oil drop discoloration.
- Splinter hemorrhages can also be present (Salomon et al. 2003).

16.6.2 Diagnosis

- Diagnosis is obvious, if they have signs of psoriasis elsewhere on the body or arthritis is present.
- About 5–10% of psoriatic patients may only have nail changes. Diagnosis becomes challenging at that time (Salomon et al. 2003).
- In toe nails, it may be difficult to rule out onychomycosis as both psoriasis and onychomycosis can have onycholysis and subungual hyperkeratosis. If coarse pitting is present along with onycholysis and subungual hyperkeratosis, it is more suggestive of psoriasis.
- A biopsy of the nail confirms the diagnosis of psoriasis (Rubin and Jellinek 2018).

16.6.3 Management

- Nail psoriasis is very resistant to topical treatments. Systemic therapies are effective in nail psoriasis.
- A 3-month trial of a combination of a topical vitamin D_3 derivative with a potent corticosteroid is done before starting systemic drugs (Hanake 2019).
- Acitretin, cyclosporine and methotrexate are the common ones used for systemic therapy (Rigopoulos et al. 2019).
- Biologic agents used for treating psoriasis include infliximab, etanercept, adalimumab and golimumab (anti-TNF alfa inhibitors); ustekinumab (IL-12/23

inhibitor); secukinumab and ixekizumab (IL-17 inhibitors); guselkumab (IL-23 inhibitor) and tofacitinib (JAK 1/3 inhibitor). Biologic agents result in more rapid and noticeable improvement when compared to other traditional systemic drugs (Hanake 2017). They also seem to have fewer side effects.

16.7 Pseudomonas Infection of the Nail

- *Pseudomonas aeruginosa* (Fig. 16.4) causes a green to brownish-black nail.

- The greenish color of the nail is very characteristic and helps in diagnosis. Confirmatory diagnosis can be provided by culture.

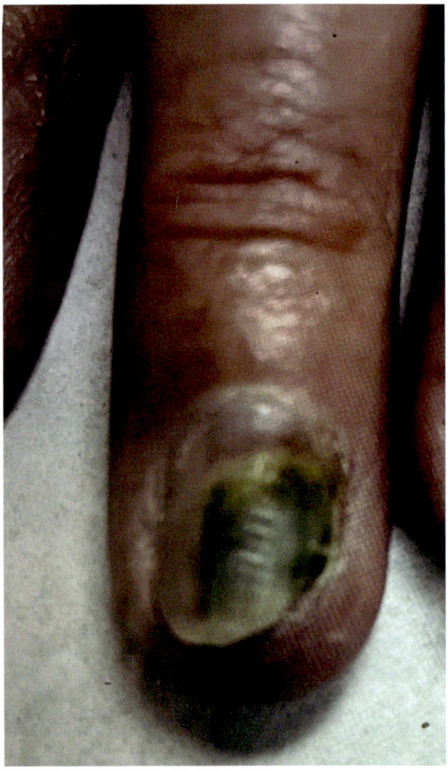

Fig. 16.4 Pseudomonas infection of the nail

16.7.1 Management

– Topical antibiotics, for instance, ciprofloxacin otic drops can be applied to the affected nail.

16.8 Paronychia

– Paronychia constitutes infection or inflammation of proximal or lateral nail folds. It can be acute (Fig. 16.5) or chronic. Inflammation of the surrounding nail folds lasting longer than 6 weeks is defined as chronic paronychia (Lee and Lipner 2022).

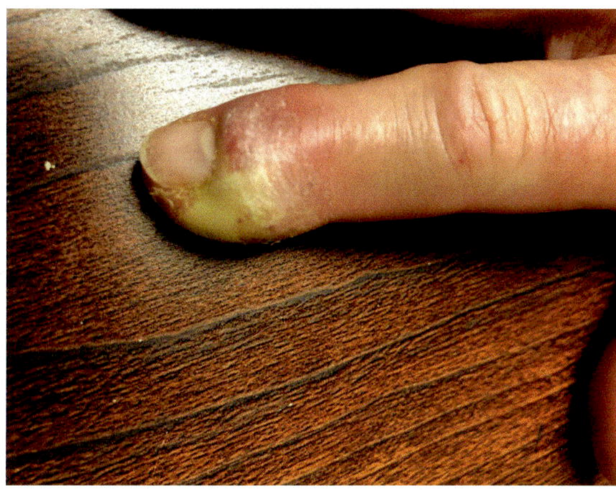

Fig. 16.5 Acute paronychia

16.8.1 Acute Paronychia

– Duration is less than 6 weeks. Usually infections are the causes.

Bacterial

– Staphylococcus is the most common cause.

– Nail fold is erythematous, swollen and warm to touch and can also have pus.

– **Management**: No abscess: Conservative therapies such as warm soaks in water or vinegar or antiseptic solutions such as povidone-iodine, chlorhexidine or burrow solution can be sufficient (Shafritz and Coppage 2014).

The affected digit should be soaked for about 10–15 min, several times a day (Rockwell 2001).

Topical antibiotics such as mupirocin or gentamicin and oral antibiotics can be added if infection persists.

If there is abscess: Incision and drainage and administration of oral antibiotics based on culture and sensitivity results. Empirical antibiotic coverage can be done with dicloxacillin, cephalexin, clindamycin or trimethoprim/sulfamethoxazole while waiting on culture and sensitivity results. The latter two are prescribed if MRSA is suspected.

16.8.2 *Chronic Paronychia*

It is usually a result of inflammation occurring due to exposure to allergens or irritants.

- Associated with damaged cuticle, either mechanical or chemical.
- The etiology is multifactorial. It is commonly due to repeated exposure to moisture and environmental irritants (Lomax et al. 2016).
- Nail fold is erythematous, sometimes scaly and sensitive, with mild swelling and an absent cuticle.
- **Management:** Avoiding irritants and exposure to excess water.

  Topical super potent steroids such as clobetasol propionate 0.05% ointment can be given.

16.9 Subungual Hematoma

- Subungual hematoma is accumulation of blood under the nail plate.
- Either direct trauma to the nail or recurrent micro traumas due to ill-fitting shoes can cause it.
- It can be differentiated from melanonychia by the fact that it does not involve the free margin of the nail plate (Hanake 2019) (Fig. 16.6).

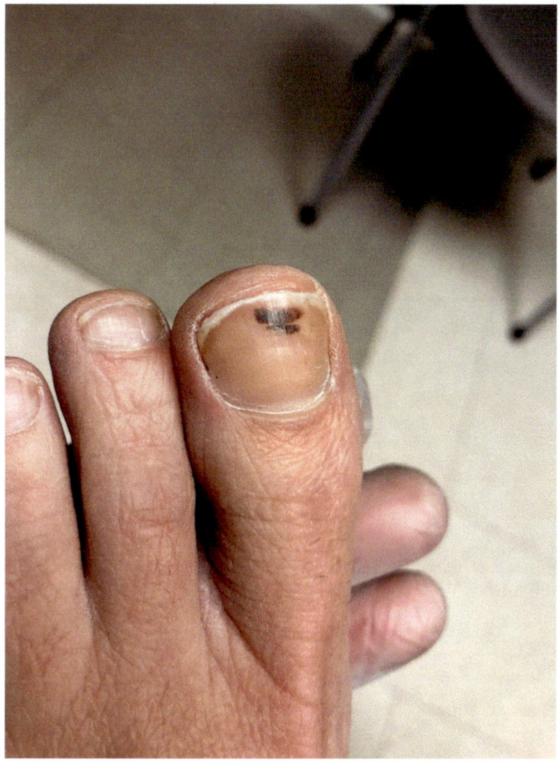

Fig. 16.6 Subungual hematoma

16.9.1 Management

- Self-limiting. No treatment needed.

16.10 Longitudinal Melanocytic Nevus (LMN) (Fig. 16.7)

- Brown or black or tan longitudinal streak within the nail plate.

- The importance of knowing this condition is because nail melanoma also can present as longitudinal melanonychia. See below for differentiating features with that of nail melanoma.

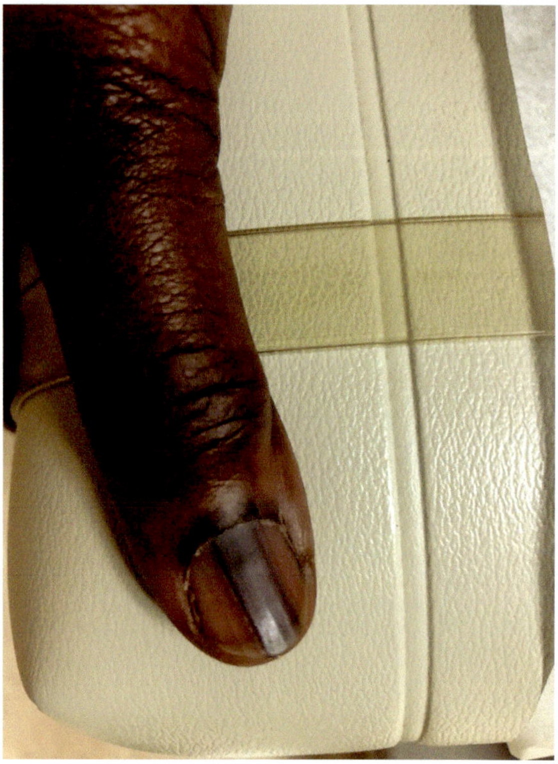

Fig. 16.7 Longitudinal melanocytic nevus

16.11 Nail Melanoma

- Although it can present as LMN, concerning signs include: asymmetry in width, varying color changes and periungual pigment extension onto proximal and/or lateral nail folds (Hutchinson sign).
- Distribution: Most often presents on thumb and first toe. Nail matrix biopsy confirms the diagnosis of nail melanoma.

Bibliography

Carley AC, Stratman EJ, Lesher JL, et al. Antimicrobial drugs. In: Bolognia J, Schaffer JV, Cerroni L, editors., et al., Dermatology. 4th ed. Amsterdam: Elsevier; 2017. p. 2231–6.

Elewski BE. Onychomycosis: pathogenesis, diagnosis, and management. Clin Microbiol Rev. 1998;11(3):415–29.

Gupta AK, Versteeg SG, Shear NH. Onychomycosis in the 21st century: an update on diagnosis, epidemiology, and treatment. J Cutan Med Surg. 2017;21(6):525–39.

Haneke E. Nail Disorders. In: Kang S et al (eds) Fitzpatrick's Dermatology, 9e. McGraw-Hill Education; 2019. https://dermatology-mhmedical-com.uab.idm.oclc.org/content.aspx?bookid=2570&sectionid=210421355

Haneke E. Nail psoriasis: clinical features, pathogenesis, differential diagnoses, and management. Psoriasis Targets Therapy. 2017;7:51–63.

LaSenna T. Patient considerations in the management of toe onychomycosis—role of efinaconazole. Patient Prefer Adherence. 2015;9:887–91.

Lee DK, Lipner SR. Optimal diagnosis and management of common nail disorders. Ann Med. 2022;54(1):694–712.

Lomax A, Thornton J, Singh D. Toenail paronychia. Foot Ankle Surg. 2016;22(4):219–23.

Preda-Naumescu A, et al. Common cutaneous infections: patient presentation, clinical course, and treatment options. Med Clin North Am. 2021;105(4):783–97. https://doi.org/10.1016/j.mcna.2021.04.012.

Rigopoulos D, Baran R, Chiheb S, Daniel CR, Di Chiacchio N, Gregoriou S, et al. Recommendations for the definition, evaluation, and treatment of nail psoriasis in adult patients with no or mild skin psoriasis: a dermatologist and nail expert group consensus. J Am Acad Dermatol. 2019;81(1):228–40.

Rockwell PG. Acute and chronic paronychia. Am Fam Phys. 2001;63(6):1113–6.

Rubin AI, Jellinek NJ, et al. Scher and Daniel's nails: diagnosis, surgery, therapy. 4th ed. Beijing: Springer; 2018.

Salomon J, Szepietowski JC, Proniewicz A. Psoriatic nails: a prospective clinical study. J Cutan Med Surg. 2003;7(4):317–21.

Shafritz AB, Coppage JM. Acute and chronic paronychia of the hand. J Am Acad Orthop Surg. 2014;22(3):165–74.

Chapter 17
Pregnancy Dermatoses

Abstract Pregnancy dermatoses consist of heterogeneous group of pruritic inflammatory dermatoses that occur exclusively during pregnancy and/or in the immediate postpartum period (Himeles and Pomeranz in Obstet Gynecol 140:679–695, 2022). The following four conditions need mention among pregnancy dermatoses from primary care scenario.

- Pemphigoid gestationis or herpes gestationis.

- Polymorphic eruption of pregnancy.

- Atopic eruption of pregnancy.

- Intrahepatic cholestasis of pregnancy.

This chapter provides an overview of the clinical manifestations of these four conditions, the potential consequence of these conditions on the outcome of the pregnancy and their management.

Keywords Herpes gestationis · Pemphigoid gestationis · Polymorphic eruption of pregnancy · Atopic eruption of pregnancy · Intrahepatic cholestasis of pregnancy · Dermatoses of pregnancy

17.1 Pemphigoid Gestationis (PG) or Herpes Gestationis

17.1.1 Clinical Features

- Manifests as intense itchy urticarial papules or plaques that progress to blisters.

- Begins on trunk, more so in the **periumbilical area,** then progresses to generalized eruption.

D. K. Yellumahanthi, *Manual of Primary Care Dermatology*,
https://doi.org/10.1007/978-3-031-68406-7_17

- Onset in 2nd or 3rd trimester. Sometimes immediately after delivery also (Himeles and Pomeranz 2022).

- About 75% of women flare at the time of delivery (Ambros-Rudolph 2011) and will require treatment.

- No known increased maternal risk (Schornick 2021).

17.1.2 Diagnosis

- Usually it requires a biopsy for histology and direct immunofluorescence (DIF). The latter is the gold standard for the diagnosis (Ambros-Rudolph 2011).

17.1.3 Fetal Risk (Himeles and Pomeranz 2022)

- Small for gestational age birth.

- Preterm delivery.

- Neonatal pemphigoid gestationis.

17.1.4 Management

- Topical steroids and oral antihistamine, (usually first generation) in mild cases. Often needs oral prednisone for more severe encounters (Ambros-Rudolph 2011).

- If not responding to steroids, Intravenous immunoglobulin or plasmapheresis may be indicated (Wiznia and Pomeranz 2019).

- For the treatment of postpartum flares of PG, rituximab, a monoclonal body, has been used (Himeles and Pomeranz 2022).

17.1.5 Prognosis

- In most cases, it resolves within a few weeks to few months postpartum; however, rarely, in some cases, it may last for years (Ambros-Rudolph 2011).

- Patients with PG can have recurrences during subsequent pregnancies. Also among about 10% of the patients, recurrences can occur while taking oral contraceptives (Himeles and Pomeranz 2022).

17.2 Polymorphic Eruption of Pregnancy

- It is the most common one among the pregnancy dermatoses (Dominguez-Serrano et al. 2019).

17.2.1 Clinical Features

- Urticarial papules or plaques with or without blisters
- **Begins on abdominal striae** (Himeles and Pomeranz 2022**) and** spreads to the rest of the trunk (**spares umbilicus unlike PG**) and then extremities.
- Onset 3rd trimester (Himeles and Pomeranz 2022).
- It does not alter maternal prognosis (Wiznia and Pomeranz 2019).

17.2.2 Fetal Risk

- None.

17.2.3 Diagnosis

Diagnosis is made based on clinical findings and history.

17.2.4 Management

- Spontaneous remission within few weeks.
- Symptomatic treatment—topical emollients, oral antihistamines. Short course of oral steroids if needed.

17.2.5 Prognosis

- Usually, it does not recur, unless in multiple pregnancies when it could recur with an early presentation (Ambros-Rudolph 2011).

17.3 Atopic Eruption of Pregnancy (AEP)

17.3.1 Clinical Features

- AEP is a disease complex comprising the previously distinct entities, prurigo of pregnancy, pruritic folliculitis of pregnancy and eczema in pregnancy (Ambros-Rudolph et al. 2006).
- Clinical picture is an overlap of eczema in pregnancy with either prurigo of pregnancy or pruritic folliculitis.

  In the former, it mainly presents as eczema with flexor and face involvement, and in the latter type, it presents mostly as discrete, itchy, excoriated papules in the extremities and trunk (Ambros-Rudolph 2011).

  Signs of eczema like xerosis are present in either type.
- Onset in most cases before 3rd trimester (Ambros-Rudolph 2011).
- There could be a history of asthma, seasonal allergies and atopy (Himeles and Pomeranz 2022).
- Not associated with any adverse maternal outcomes (Kurien et al. 2024).

17.3.2 Fetal Risk

- None.

17.3.3 Diagnosis

- Diagnosis is made based on clinical findings and history.

17.3.4 Management

- Topical emollients or topical moderate potent steroids or oral antihistamines help with symptomatic treatment. A short course of systemic steroids may be required for severe or recalcitrant cases (Ambros-Rudolph 2011).

17.4 Intrahepatic Cholestasis of Pregnancy (ICP)

17.4.1 Clinical Features

- No primary skin lesion noted. Severe pruritus is the only initial symptom in most cases. Secondary Excoriations and excoriated papules can be present due to scratching (Schornick 2021).

- Generalized distribution.

- Systemic symptoms such as fatigue, anorexia, nausea may be present.

- Jaundice may or may not be present.

- Onset in 3rd trimester.

- Although maternal outcomes are usually favorable, postpartum hemorrhage can occur in severe cases due to vitamin K depletion (Wiznia and Pomeranz 2019). These patients can also develop gallbladder disease or cholelithiasis in future (Wiznia and Pomeranz 2019).

17.4.2 Fetal Risk

- Fetal risk includes fetal death and premature births (Schornick 2021).

17.4.3 Diagnosis

- Elevated serum bile acids (> 11 μm per liter).

17.4.4 Management

- Resolves within 2–4 weeks of delivery (Schornick 2021).

- Ursodeoxycholic acid is the treatment of choice.

- There is mixed data in the literature regarding early delivery with most seem to be recommending early induction of labor, commonly at 36 weeks of gestation (Bicocca et al. 2018; Lo et al. 2014).

17.4.5 Prognosis

- Patients with ICP can manifest it in subsequent pregnancies (Himeles and Pomeranz 2022).

Bibliography

Ambros-Rudolph CM. Dermatoses of pregnancy—clues to diagnosis, fetal risk and therapy. Ann Dermatol. 2011;23(3):265.

Ambros-Rudolph CM, Müllegger RR, Vaughan-Jones SA, et al. The specific dermatoses of pregnancy revisited and reclassified: results of a retrospective two-center study on 505 pregnant patients. J Am Acad Dermatol. 2006;54:395–404.

Bicocca MJ, Sperling JD, Chauhan SP. Intrahepatic cholestasis of pregnancy: review of six national and regional guidelines. Euro J Obstetrics Gynecol Reprod Biol. 2018;231:180–7. Available from https://www.sciencedirect.com/science/article/pii/S0301211518310571.

Dominguez-Serrano AJ, Quiroga-Garza A, Jacobo-Baca G, De La Fuente-Villarreal D, Gonzalez-Ramirez RA, Vazquez-Barragan MA, Guzman-Lopez A, Elizondo-Omaña RE, Guzman-Lopez S. Polymorphic eruption of pregnancy in Mexico. Int J Dermatol. 2019;58(3):259–62.

Himeles JR, Pomeranz MK. Recognizing, diagnosing, and managing pregnancy dermatoses. Obstet Gynecol. 2022;140(4):679–95.

Kurien G, Carlson K, Badri T. Dermatoses of pregnancy. In: StatPearls. Treasure Island: StatPearls Publishing; 2024. PMID: 28613614.

Lo JO, Shaffer BL, Allen AJ, Little SE, Cheng YW, Caughey AB. Intrahepatic cholestasis of pregnancy and timing of delivery. J Matern Fetal Neonatal Med. 2014;28(18):2254–8.

Schornick J. Dermatoses of pregnancy. In: Waldman RA, Grant-Kels JM, editors. Dermatology for the primary care provider. Elsevier, Inc.; 2021.

Wiznia LE, Pomeranz M. Skin changes and diseases in pregnancy. In: Kang S, Amagai M, Bruckner AL, Enk AH, Margolis DJ, McMichael AJ, Orringer JS, editors. Fitzpatrick's dermatology, 9e. McGraw-Hill Education; 2019.

Chapter 18
Skin Biopsies and Cryosurgery

Abstract Skin biopsies and cryosurgery are the common procedures that are done in primary care. Mainly three types of skin biopsies are performed: shave biopsy; punch biopsy and excisional biopsy. Cryosurgery is a kind of treatment modality that is popularly employed for the purpose of destruction of benign, premalignant and malignant skin lesions. Liquid nitrogen, which boils at – 196 °C (– 320.8°F), is the most common cryogen used in cryosurgery. In this chapter, we will briefly discuss about cryosurgery and common biopsy techniques.

Keywords Shave biopsy · Punch biopsy · Excisional biopsy · Cryotherapy · Elliptical biopsy · Skin biopsy

18.1 Skin Biopsy

Mainly three types of skin biopsies are performed.

- Shave biopsy.
- Punch biopsy.
- Excisional biopsy using an elliptical excision.

18.1.1 Shave Biopsy

- It is usually appropriate for those lesions that are raised or pedunculated.
- At the site of biopsy, local anesthesia is provided by either with lidocaine or with lidocaine and epinephrine. The injection is given either intradermally or subcutaneous. If administered by former route, at the overlying skin, a raised blanching wheel would be noticed.

D. K. Yellumahanthi, *Manual of Primary Care Dermatology*,
https://doi.org/10.1007/978-3-031-68406-7_18

- For non-pedunculated or flatter lesions, if local anesthetic is administered intradermally, the raised wheel can give enough space for a shave biopsy to be performed (Jarell and Schalock 2012).

- One does not have to wait long after administering local anesthesia to start the procedure. In author's experience, about 5 min after the administration of anesthesia was adequate.

- Derma blade is the common instrument used for shave biopsy. Razor blade can be used as well. To begin with, first, one has to stabilize the skin lesion by using the index finger and thumb of the non-dominant hand. Later, derma blade (or razor blade) is held parallel to the skin surface so that it gets to the upper dermis level, and in a gradual see-saw motion, the skin lesion is removed from its base. If the skin lesion does not get separated automatically, a toothed forceps can be used to separate the skin lesion from the base of the skin surface.

- No sutures need to be placed. Minimal bleeding can be controlled with measures such as application of silver nitrate or applying pressure.

- Biopsy specimen is placed in the container containing formalin to be transported to the lab.

18.1.2 Punch Biopsy

- This is another commonly used technique. Although several size punches are available, 4 mm is the most commonly used one and usually it provides adequate tissue for the pathologist.

- The initial steps of punch biopsy up to administration of local anesthesia are similar to shave biopsy. Traction also needs to be obtained in a similar way so that the lesion can be stabilized. Instead of using the derma blade, instrument 'punch' is used.

  Punch is placed on the skin lesion such that the whole diameter of the punch lies on the skin lesion of interest. Then slowly the punch is twisted and at the same time pressed so that the punch makes its way into the skin lesion. When the punch has penetrated enough depth into the skin lesion, the twisting process can be stopped and punch can be lifted from the skin lesion. The material of the skin lesion equivalent to the diameter of the punch comes out along with the punch when the punch is retracted from the skin lesion. If it does not happen automatically, forceps and scissors can be used to complete the process of getting the biopsy material out.

- 4 mm punch biopsy sites need not always have to be sutured. If needed, one or two interrupted sutures can be placed using prolene or any such material. The time of removal of the sutures varies as per the body site. While facial sutures need to be removed within a week, those at other places can be left for about two weeks (Jarell and Schalock 2012).

- For both shave and punch biopsies, clean field is sufficient. The provider performing the procedure only needs to have a clean gloves and not necessarily sterile gloves (Jarell and Schalock 2012).

18.1.3 Excisional Biopsy Using an Elliptical Excision

- During the excisional biopsy, as the name states, the whole skin lesion is usually removed.

- Unlike the shave and punch biopsies, elliptical excision requires sterile field (Jarell and Schalock 2012).

- A 15 G scalpel, surgical skin marker, tooted forceps, iris scissors, needle holder and suture material are needed. Care should be taken to make sure electrocautery, or similar equipment is available for hemostasis.

- Before the anesthesia is given, the borders of the ellipse are marked using a surgical skin marker. Ellipse should include both the skin lesion and the desired margin.

- After the ellipse is marked, using a 15G scalpel first an indentation is made along the line of the ellipse. A 15 G blade should be held vertically to the skin surface initially, and it should start at the apex of the ellipse. After piercing to the subcutaneous level at the apex, the scalpel is tilted such that it can cut through the margin of the ellipse to the other apex. Similar maneuver needs to be done at the other margin of the ellipse as well. Once the ellipse was cut to subcutaneous tissue all along its borders, using forceps and scalpel or scissors, the ellipse can be cut away from the surrounding skin in a single piece.

- The material taken out is placed in formalin to be sent to the lab.

- Hemostasis is secured with electrocautery.

- If the edges needed to be undermined before suturing, it can be done.

- Skin can be placed either in layers or in one layer. If subcuticular stiches need to be placed, an absorbable suture material such as vicryl is used. Skin sutures are done either with interrupted or continuous. Usually non-absorbable material is used for the skin. Sutures are removed at the appropriate time as was mentioned above during the 'punch biopsy' section.

18.2 Cryosurgery

- Cryosurgery is a kind of treatment modality that is popularly employed for the purpose of destruction of benign, premalignant and malignant skin lesions.

- Liquid nitrogen, which boils at − 196 °C (− 320.8°F), is the most common cryogen used in cryosurgery (Prohaska and Jan 2024).

- Selective necrosis of targeted tissues/skin lesion while making sure that the surrounding tissue is uninjured is the goal of cryosurgery (Jarell and Schalock 2012).

- Although there are various techniques that can be used to accomplish this objective, among all those, timed spot freezing is the common one as it allows greater standardization of delivery of liquid nitrogen (Andrews 2004).

- For timed spot freezing, a handheld cryo gun/canister is often the equipment that is used. It has different probes of various sizes which can be appropriately used depending upon factors such as the type of skin lesion, the thickness of the lesion and sometimes also based on its location.

- The handheld spray cryo gun is usually placed at a distance of 1–1.5 inch away from the skin lesion that is intended to be sprayed (Andrews 2004).

- The patient should be placed in such a way that the skin lesion is not at a very high level so that while spraying, the cryo canister/gun does not need to be tilted up. The spraying should be done aiming at the center of the lesion. The spraying should be done until an ice ball is formed covering both the lesion and a desired margin.

- The size of the desired margin of the ice ball depends mainly on whether the lesion is benign or malignant and also on the thickness of the lesion. The usual margins' range is from 1 to 2 mm for the benign lesions, 2–3 mm for premalignant lesions and about 5 mm for malignant lesions (Andrews 2004).

- Once the desired size of the ice ball is formed, spraying needs to be continued maintaining the same size of the ice ball for a given length of time which is called 'Freeze time'. The freeze time varies as per the nature of the targeted skin lesion.

- After the lesion is sprayed for the given length of freeze time, the lesion needed to be completely thawed before it is resprayed if it required two freeze-thaw cycles. The disappearance of ice ball is often an indicator that the lesion is thawed. It is also prudent to make sure that patient is relieved of any discomfort from the first freeze thaw cycle before it is resprayed.

- For pedunculated lesions such as skin tags, instead of the spray technique, grasping the skin tag with a cryo tweezer may be more convenient.

- The conditions for which cryosurgery is commonly employed include:

  Warts, actinic keratosis, seborrheic keratosis, molluscum contagiosum, skin tags and non-melanoma skin cancers such as basal cell cancer and squamous cell cancer in situ (Prohaska and Jan 2024).

- Contraindications for cryosurgery include:

  Melanoma, lesions for which tissue pathology is required, lesions where diagnosis is uncertain, Raynaud's disease and other conditions where exposure to cold temperatures are hazardous.

Below is a list of some common condition, their suggested freeze times and the number of freeze-thaw cycles required (Table 18.1).

Table 18.1 Some common skin conditions, their freeze time and number of freeze-thaw cycles required for cryotherapy

Skin lesion	Freeze time	Number of freeze-thaw cycles
Warts (Primary Care Dermatology Society)	10–30 seconds	Usually one. For plantar warts two
Skin tag (Andrews 2004)	5 seconds	One
Seborrheic Keratosis (Primary Care Dermatology Society)	5–30 seconds	One
Actinic Keratosis (Primary Care Dermatology Society)	5–10 seconds	One
BCC (Collins et al. 2019)	40–90 seconds based on factors such as the type, size and location	Two
SCC in situ (Bowen's disease) (Primary Care Dermatology Society)	15–30 seconds	One

– Local anesthesia with lidocaine can be done an hour before the procedure to minimize the pain associated with freezing when longer freeze time is required such as in cases of BCC.

– Adverse effects include pain and burning/itching at the site of application, erythema lasting hours to few days and crusting for 1–2 weeks. A blister can form at the site of application. Patients need to be cautioned about it. Blister does not have to be treated unless it ruptures. In which case, any antiseptic cream such as polysporin can be used to prevent secondary bacterial infection. Hypopigmentation and alopecia at the site of cryotherapy can also occur.

Bibliography

Andrews MD. Cryosurgery for common skin conditions. Am Fam Physician [Internet]. 2004;69(10):2365–72. Available from: https://www.aafp.org/pubs/afp/issues/2004/0515/p2365.html

Collins A, Savas J, Doerfler L. Nonsurgical treatments for nonmelanoma skin cancer. Dermatol Clin. 2019;37(4):435–41.

Jarell A, Schalock PC. Procedures in dermatologic diagnosis and therapy. In: Schalock PC, Hsu JTS, Arndt KA, editors. Lippincott's primary care dermatology. Lippincott Williams & Wilkins; 2012.

Cryosurgery (also known as cryotherapy) [Internet]. Primary Care Dermatology Society. Available from: https://www.pcds.org.uk/clinical-guidance/cryosurgery

Prohaska J, Jan AH. Cryotherapy in dermatology. In: StatPearls [Internet]. Treasure Island (FL): n Publishing; 2024. Available from: https://www-ncbi-nlm-nih-gov.uab.idm.oclc.org/books/NBK482319/ [Updated 2023 Sep 15].

Index

D. K. Yellumahanthi, *Manual of Primary Care Dermatology*,
https://doi.org/10.1007/978-3-031-68406-7

MIX
Papier aus verantwortungsvollen Quellen
Paper from responsible sources
FSC® C105338
www.fsc.org
FSC

If you have any concerns about our products,
you can contact us on
ProductSafety@springernature.com

In case Publisher is established outside the EU,
the EU authorized representative is:
Springer Nature Customer Service Center GmbH
Europaplatz 3, 69115 Heidelberg, Germany

Printed by Libri Plureos GmbH
in Hamburg, Germany